ANORECTAL
DISEASE IN AIDS

ANORECTAL
DISEASE IN AIDS

Edited by
T G Allen-Mersh
and L Gottesman

Edward Arnold

A division of Hodder & Stoughton

LONDON   MELBOURNE   AUCKLAND

© 1991 TG Allen-Mersh and L Gottesman

First published in Great Britain 1991

British Library Cataloguing in Publication Data
Allen-Mersh, T. G.
  Anorectal disease in AIDS.
  I. Title II. Gottesman, L.
  616.97

  ISBN 0 340 54643 3

Typeset in Linotron Palatino by
Rowland Phototypesetting Limited, Bury St Edmunds, Suffolk
Printed and bound in Great Britain for Edward Arnold, a division of
Hodder and Stoughton Limited, Mill Road, Dunton Green,
Sevenoaks, Kent TN13 2YA by
Butler and Tanner Limited, Frome, Somerset

Preface

The HIV epidemic has brought new challenges for the colon-rectal surgeon. Anorectal disorders—particularly venereological diseases—were previously commoner among homosexual than non-homosexual males, but the association with immune-deficiency has resulted in both new diseases and novel presentations of previously recognized conditions. While a nihilistic approach to treatment of these conditions is inappropriate, management must be tempered with an awareness of the natural history of HIV disease.

This book includes contributions on many aspects of anorectal disease in the HIV-positive male. The contributors have learnt about these conditions from their own clinical practice as colorectal surgeons or AIDS physicians during the past decade of the HIV epidemic. There is much that can be done to relieve anorectal symptoms in these patients. We hope this book provides a logical approach to evaluation and treatment.

It is a pleasure to acknowledge the generous support of Regent Hospital Products, manufacturers of Biogel powder-free surgeons' gloves, in subsidizing the printing costs of this book as part of their contribution to medical education.

TG Allen-Mersh
Lester Gottesman
1991

Contents

List of contributors

TG Allen-Mersh MD, FRCS, Department of Surgery Westminster Hospital, London, England

A Borcich MD, Department of Medicine, St Luke's–Roosevelt Hospital Center; and the College of Physicians and Surgeons, Columbia University, New York, USA

GM Connolly MB, MRCPI, Department of Gastroenterology, Westminster Hospital, London, England

TI Davidson ChM, MRCP, FRCS, Department of Surgery, Westminster Hospital, London, England

BS Gingold MD, FACS, Department of Surgery, St Vincent's Hospital, New York City, NY, USA

L Gottesman MD, Division of Colon Rectal Surgery, St Luke's–Roosevelt Hospital Center, New York City, NY, USA

DA Hawkins BSc, MRCP, Department of Genito-Urinary Medicine and Venereology, St. Stephen's Clinic and Westminster Hospital, London, England

DP Kotler MD, GI Division, St Luke's–Roosevelt Hospital Center, New York City, NY, USA

CE Metroka MD, Division of Hematology–Oncology, St Luke's–Roosevelt Hospital Center; and the College of Physicians and Surgeons, Columbia University, New York City, NY, USA

AJG Miles FRCS, Department of Surgery, Westminster Hospital, London, England

JMA Northover MS, FRCS, ICRF Colorectal Unit, St Mark's Hospital, London, England

J. Rainey ChM, FRCS(Ed.), Department of Surgery, St John's Hospital at Howden, West Lothian, Scotland

WP Schecter MD, University of California, San Francisco, CA, USA

JH Scholefield MS, FRCS, ICRF Colorectal Unit, St Mark's Hospital, London, England

ME Soler MD, Division of Colon Rectal Surgery, St Luke's–Roosevelt Hospital Center, New York City, NY, USA

A Vallejo MD, Division of Radiation Oncology, St Luke's–Roosevelt Hospital Center, New York City, NY, USA

SD Wexner MD, Staff Colorectal Surgeon Residency Program Director. Anorectal Physiology Laboratory, Cleveland Director Clinic Florida, FL, USA

BACKGROUND

1

Biology of HIV infection
Anthony Borcich and Donald P Kotler

Introduction

The anorectal junction is a complex area both anatomically and physiologically. The epithelial lining layers include skin and rectal mucosa plus a transitional zone in the anal canal. The tissues underlying the skin and mucosa also differ. The mucosal and cutaneous compartments face different local external environments. For example, the rectal mucosa is in contact with an anaerobic environment while atmospheric gases are in contact with perianal skin. The immune defences of the areas also differ. The immune defences of the skin are part of the systemic immune system while the immune defenses in the rectum are part of the mucosal immune system.

The integument is an effective barrier to the penetration of foreign materials. The layers of keratinized superficial epithelium make the skin non-wettable and virtually impervious to penetration by bacteria. The integument also is an immunologically active organ. The basal layer of the epidermis contains immunocompetent Langerhan's cells (also called dendritic cells) that phagocytose particulate foreign antigens. These antigens are partially digested in the cell, then expressed at the cell membrane, where they are 'presented' to T lymphocytes, which can become sensitized. Sensitized cells migrate from the skin through the lymphatics to peripheral lymph nodes, where proliferation and differentiation occur by well-described mechanisms to produce an immune reponse [1].

The lining of the mucous membranes differs considerably from skin. It presents a weak physical barrier to penetration by viruses, bacteria or other pathogenic agents. Functionally, it is a lipid membrane of no more strength than a droplet of oil on water. However, it is a continuous lipid membrane, interrupted only by the spaces between epithelial cells (tight junctions), so that penetration by water-soluble materials is limited. Specialized transport proteins on small intestinal and colonic epithelial cell membranes allow for the highly selective binding and uptake of materials into the cell. The selective permeability of the intestinal epithelium is extremely important in preventing the entry of potentially toxic metabolites and other materials that are ingested or excreted in bile.

The integrity of the fragile mucous membranes is maintained by a variety of immunologic and non-immunologic factors. The mucous membranes are defended by an immune system whose functions are distinct from systemic immunity [2]. While there is a common embryologic heritage, the systemic and mucosal immune systems function, in large part, independently in the body. This is accomplished through the expression of certain receptors on the cell membranes of mucosal mononuclear cells that recognize receptors in vascular endothelium (high endothelial venules) in the mucous membranes. Receptor interactions explain the results of elegantly performed experiments in which labelled mucosal lymphocytes, given intravenously, migrated specifically to mucous membranes, and especially to the areas from which the cells were derived [3]. The results of these studies also indicate that there is a common mucosal immune system with direct communication between the various mucous membrane compartments [4].

The mucosal immune system is composed of focal and diffuse collections of cells. Lymphoid follicles occur either in aggregates, such as in the tonsils and the Peyer's patches, or as single structures as in the rectum. There are as many as 12 lymphoid follicles per square centimeter in the colon and rectum [5]. The epithelium overlying mucosal lymphoid follicles contains specialized cells (M cells). These cells lack microvilli and an overlying coat of mucus, and allow penetration of particulate antigens [6]. The antigens that pass through M cells are phagocytosed by macrophages in the mucosal lymphoid follicles and presented to T lymphocytes, which direct subsequent B lymphocyte development. The lymphoid follicles, thus, are the site of initial antigen recognition and lymphoid activation. Activated cells subsequently migrate to distant sites, especially the mesenteric lymph nodes, and differentiate before returning to the intestine. Several studies have documented the complex trafficking of activated mucosal T lymphocytes.

The layers of the intestinal mucosa contain a diversity of diffusely localized, immunologically active cells. The epithelial layer contains several cell types. The T suppressor lymphocyte (CD8+) is the major cell type found [7]. The CD8+ cells in the epithelium appear to mediate suppression rather than cytotoxicity, as is the case in other compartments of the body. Intraepithelial macrophages are the other important cell type. Occasional mast cells or eosinophils may be seen in normal epithelium. On the other hand, the presence of neutrophils in the epithelium is indicative of a pathologic process.

T lymphocytes are scattered diffusely in the lamina propria with the proportion of helper T lymphocytes to suppressor T lymphocytes being about the same as found in peripheral blood (1.5–2.0) [8]. The T lymphocytes perform regulatory functions in the lamina propria. About 10% of the lymphocytes in the lamina propria are B lymphocytes. Plasma cells are another important constituent of the cell population and are found predominantly in a band about 200 microns thick located just below the surface of the epithelium. Macrophages are the major form of phagocytic cell in the lamina propria. However, eosinophils and mast cells also are found in mucosal biopsies from healthy individuals [9]. As is the case in the epithelial layer, extravascular neutrophils are not a normal constituent of the lamina propria.

The antibody system in the intestine is specialized in that most of the antibody produced is of the IgA variety [10]. IgA differs from IgG in that two molecules of IgA are linked together by a peptide called a J-piece to form a dimer. The IgA antibody functions mainly in the intestinal lumen rather than in the tissue compartment, where it binds to relevant antigens and prevents them from interacting with and penetrating the epithelial cell membrane. This function is termed 'antigen exclusion'. The IgA is actively secreted from the crypt epithelial cell, which transports it from the lamina propria to the lumen. A glycosolated peptide called 'secretory component', which protects the antibody from degradation, is added to the antibody during transepithelial transport. Hepatic bile also contains IgA antibody. The relative contribution of hepatic IgA secretion to total IgA secretion varies between species.

Delayed hypersensitivity reactions in the mucous membranes, which are mediated and regulated by T lymphocytes, are very similar to reactions in other compartments of the body. Under the direction of the helper T lymphocytes, various classes of cytotoxic cells—including macrophages, natural killer cells and lymphokine-activated killer cells—recognize and destroy infected cells or cells that demonstrate malignant potential.

Mucosal immunity is a well-coordinated and highly regulated system. Despite its location in approximation to high concentrations of potential pathogens, the mucosa itself is relatively uninflamed. A finely balanced system of immune suppression and activation (contrasuppression) limits the intensity and extent of an immune reaction to its most efficient size and duration [11]. This balance limits unnecessary damage and dysfunction to the gut, which is important considering its vital roles of nutrient and water absorption.

Mucosal immune function is also integrated with systemic immunity in several ways. One such integration involves the active suppression of systemic immune responses to antigens to which the mucosal tissues have previously been immunized (tolerance) [12] The presence of tolerance limits the ability to respond adversely to the introduction of an innocuous foreign antigen, such as a food antigen, into the body.

Other, non-immunological factors promote the defense of the GI tract especially in the anorectal region. The secretion of mucins plays several roles [13]. Mucus act as a lubricant to aid the passage of solid materials. This gel-like material is a diffusion barrier for particulate materials but does not affect the diffusion of soluble materials such as water, ions or the products of intraluminal digestion. Mucins also contain receptors for IgA and for other proteins, such as lysozyme, which deter penetration by bacteria. There also are receptors occupied by non pathogenic bacteria which help prevent colonization by pathogenic bacteria.

Intestinal motility is not an important component of the defense of the rectum, in the absence of pathological states such as constipation, though peristalisis is an important factor in maintaining low intraluminal bacterial counts in the upper intestine. Anti-infective properties of pancreatic and biliary secretions likewise do not play a significant role in the defense of the anorectal region, with the exception of a generalized increase in susceptibility to enteric pathogens in patients with diminished gastric acid secretion.

The normal colonic flora plays an important role in the body's economy and contributes to the defense of the anorectal region. The colonic flora includes a wide variety of bacteria in varying proportions and is remarkably stable over long periods of time [14]. The bacteria serve physiologic functions, such as the fermentation of some unabsorbed fiber as well as malabsorbed carbohydrates to short-chain fatty acids, which can diffuse into the bloodstream. Short-chain fatty acids can be converted to metabolizable compounds so that a substantial fraction of the energy from malabsorbed carbohydrates can be salvaged. They may be an important energy source for the epithelial cells [15].

The normal flora also serves a defensive function for the body by suppressing the proliferation of potential pathogenic agents, even in the presence of colonization. This is well illustrated by *Clostridium difficile* which can be isolated from the intestines of many healthy people. The growth of *C. difficile* may be inhibited by bacterial products. When broad-spectrum antibiotics are administered, colonic bacterial counts diminish markedly. The growth of *C. difficile* may then increase owing to the loss of inhibition and result in sufficient toxin formation to produce the well-recognized syndrome of pseudomembraneous colitis [16].

Epidemiology

Initially described in 1981 as an acquired deficiency of immune function occurring in promiscuous homosexual males [17,18], the Acquired Immunodeficiency Syndrome (AIDS) was soon recognized to occur in parenteral drug users, hemophiliacs, heterosexual men and women, children of mothers with the syndrome, and recipients of blood products [19]. The disease has spread rapidly worldwide, as evidence by an initial doubling of the number of US cases every six months; the present rate is half this figure. Serologic studies, developed after the recognition and isolation of the human immunodeficiency virus type 1 (HIV-1), the etiologic agent for the illness, indicate a high rate of infection in several population groups, and the rate of conversion from seropostive asymptomatic to eventual clinical AIDS is believed to approach 100%. In 1986, for example, 70% of homosexual males in San Francisco and 60% of parenteral drug users in New York City were seropositive. While the rate of new infections (seroconversion) in the homosexual community has slowed, disease spread among heterosexuals, especially in ghetto neighborhoods, is unchecked. The prospects for a progressively increasing caseload is of great concern to health care planners as AIDS becomes a larger burden on health care resources.

Early epidemiologic observations implicating parenteral and mucous membrane routes of exposure suggested an infectious etiologic agent. Various bodily secretions, such as semen or breast milk, are capable of transmitting virus, but disease spread via casual contact, as occurs among household members, is rare [20,21]. Indeed, HIV may be particularly concentrated in semen, and transmission via receptive intercourse, anal more than vaginal, is relatively efficient. It is not known if mucous membrane disruption is necessary for transmission, nor if the virus requires an intermediate vector, such as an infected lymphocyte.

Virology

The human immunodeficiency virus type 1 (HIV-1), the etiologic agent of AIDS, was isolated almost simultaneously by several laboratories from patients with AIDS and subjects at risk for the disease [22,23]. Other retroviruses, which are distinct from HIV-1 but which produce clinical immunodeficiency, have since been isolated [24]. HIV is a member of the family of lentiviruses (slow viruses), producing clinical disease after a long latent period. HIV-1 is a genetically distant relative of the other disease-producing human retroviruses, HTLV-I and HTLV-II [25], and is more closely related to certain non-human retroviruses that cause chronic progressive degenerative diseases, such as simian immune deficiency syndrome [26].

Retroviruses are RNA-coded viruses that contain reverse transcriptase, an enzyme which transcribes RNA into DNA. Retroviral infection may be latent, in which DNA is integrated into host genome, or productive, where RNA replication and virus assembly occurs. Viral replication does not occur in latently infected cells, although viral genes may affect host cell function. An important aspect of infection by HIV and other retroviruses is that the number of productively infected cells is very low relative to the number of latently infected cells. This results in few virally infected cells being 'seen' by the host's immune system and helps explain why the immune response is ineffective in clearing the infection.

HIV is an obligate intracellular pathogen, and HIV genome or antigens have been identified in several cell types. The CD4+ lymphocyte (helper T lymphocyte) was the first cell target to be identified. It is vulnerable to infection by HIV as it carries a high density of CD4 receptors on the cell membrane. Normally involved in antigen recognition in association with the major histocompatibility class II antigens, CD4 is also an attachment site for HIV [27]. Macrophages also are an important cellular reservoir for HIV infection [28]. HIV genome and/or protein antigens also have been found in a variety of other immunologically active cells as well as neural cells, kidney cells and others. Cellular reservoirs for HIV in the GI tract include lymphocytes and macrophages in the lamna propria [29]. Some authors have also found evidence of HIV in epithelial cells and intraepithelial mononuclear cells [30].

Studies from several laboratories have shown that the HIV genome is prone to mutations [31]. There are several potential consequences of such genomic variation. Mutations in the gene coding for the viral envelope protein (gp 120) may result in subtle variations in the primary and tertiary structures of this protein, which could affect the binding of virus to target cells. For example, different isolates of HIV are variously cytopathic for CD4+ lymphocytes and macrophages [32]. Such mutations also could affect the susceptibility to antiviral immunity. Mutations in the viral regulatory genes may affect the virulence of the viral infection, leading to enhanced

viral cytotoxicity [33]. Mutations of the genes coding for viral DNA polymerase or other proteins may confer resistance to antiviral therapies [34].

The outcome of cellular viral infection is related to factors besides the
intrinsic virulence of the virus. Viral production *in vitro* may be modulated
by several agents. Viral interactions have been shown to occur between HIV
and other viruses, especially herpes viruses, whose products increase HIV
protein production through effects on a specific portion of the genome, the
tat or transactivating gene [35]. Virus production also can be modulated
through the effects of specific cytokines such as interleukin-2, tumor necrosis factor or others, which act at a different portion of the HIV genome, the
NF kappa B region [36]. The latter processes may be quite significant since
cytokine release may occur from a variety of stimuli. HIV reactivation from
cytokines could explain how HIV infection might be promoted by inflammation due to unrelated infections, such as venereal diseases.

Immune dysfunction in AIDS

Immune dysfunction occurs as a direct or indirect result of HIV infection.
The most significant feature of HIV infection is depletion of CD4+ T helper
cells. The degree of immune dysfunction roughly parallels CD4+ lymphocyte depletion. Cell death occurs as a result of viral cytopathy or through
other mechanisms, including immunologic destruction of virally infected
cells [37]. Other aspects of the disease process which promote immune
deficiency include the destruction of dendritic cells, damage to the thymus,
and immune dysregulation, which results in the production of auto-
antibodies and of immune complexes with persistent complement
activation.

The CD4+ lymphocyte is the coordinator for integrated immune function,
exerting its effects through the production of specific cytokines [38]. Helper
lymphocytes interact with B lymphocytes, macrophages and killer cells to
produce a multifaceted attack upon an invading pathogen. Depletion or
functional impairment of CD4+ lymphocytes, thus, has widespread deleterious effects on immunity, including defects in antibody production, delayed hypersensitivity reactions, and macrophage functions. The defects
include diminished surveillance against the development of neoplasms.

Mucosal immunity in AIDS has received little attention. It is likely that
homologous defects occur in the mucosal and systemic immune systems,
though it is not clear that the statuses of cells in peripheral blood accurately
reflect the situation in tissue-bound cells. However, studies of mucosal
lymphocyte subpopulations using immunohistochemical techniques
demonstrated equivalent decreases in the helper T cell population in blood
and intestinal mucosa in patients with ARC and AIDS [39]. The number of
killer cells was preserved in the intestine of AIDs patients [39], however,
though qualitative and quantitative killer cell deficiency in peripheral blood
has been demonstrated repeatedly [40]. Secretory immune deficiency occurs
in patients with AIDS. Studies have shown a depletion of IgA containing
plasma cells in jejunal and rectal biopsies from AIDS patients as well as a
decrease in salivary IgA secretion [41]. Clinical observations of patients with

cytomegalovirus and *Mycobacterium avium intracellulare* infections of the intestine indicate that delayed hypersensitivity reactions are blunted in the intestines of AIDS patients. The occurrence of Kaposi's sarcoma and B cell lymphoma in the GI tracts of AIDS patients imply that surveillance against the development of neoplasms also is adversely affected in AIDS.

Clinical consequences of the immune dysfunction

Several types of disease processes affect the anorectum of HIV-infected persons. These disease processes include opportunistic infections such as are found in other regions of the body, as well as typical and atypical presentations of diseases that also can affect immune competent persons. The clinical management of anorectal diseases in HIV-infected persons usually involves tissue biopsy and/or culture, which are rquired for diagnostic certainty and to exclude the possibility of multiple pathogens.

It is convenient to subdivide the lesions affecting the anorectum into ulcers, masses, warts, infections, and vascular (hemorrhoidal) lesions. These lesions will be discussed in greater detail in other chapters.

The incidence of neoplasms is markedly increased in AIDS. As there is approximately a 100-fold increase in the incidence of anogenital cancers in renal transplant recipients maintained under chronic immunosuppression, it is not surprising that the defects in cell-mediated immunity that occur in AIDS also lead to an increased incidence of neoplasms. A viral etiology in transplant-associated cancers has been speculated, which is consistent with the concept of diminished immune surveillance against developing neoplasms.

Protein-energy malnutrition is a common and serious complication of AIDS [42]. The magnitude of depletion may determine the timing of death from wasting illnesses [43]. The relative contributions of body cell mass and body fat depletion vary in different patients. The development of malnutrition is multifactorial and includes alterations in nutrient intake, absorption and metabolism. The occurrence of such alterations is usually due to identifiable causes, which are potentially treatable. HIV itself may play a direct role in the promotion of body mass depletion. The development of malnutrition has important ramifications for immune function, cognitive function and 'quality of life', in particular. There also are larger, societal issues relevant to AIDS, and chronic disease in general. As in other diseases, malnutrition in AIDS may affect the ability of a patient to respond to specific therapies, such as surgery [44].

The major goal of nutritional therapy in AIDS is repletion of body mass. Recent studies have demonstrated the ability of AIDS patients to replete body mass as a result of enteral or parenteral therapies [45, 46], or to respond favorably to appetite stimulants [47]. Nutritional repletion also may occur when disease complications are successfully treated [48].

Surgery of anorectal conditions in AIDS

Discussion of the role of surgery in the therapy of anorectal and other complications in HIV-infected patients is complex. The controversies surrounding the application of surgical therapies includes not only the risk to the patient, but also the risks to the surgical team. Many studies have documented transient adverse effects of anesthesia and surgery on immunological function [49]. The outcome of surgical procedures is also affected by the underlying disease state, the stage of HIV infection, concomitant diseases, and nutritional status, as well as other factors. Little formal study has been given to the topic and the published results represent unccontrolled observations. Several reports indicate a high rate of poor outcomes of anorectal surgical procedures [49–51]. However, other studies have demonstrated that HIV-infected patients may benefit greatly from surgical therapies—for example, splenectomy for severe, unresponsive thrombocytopenia [52]. In our experience, many patients with AIDS have recovered after surgery for potentially life-threatening conditions, such as perforated duodenal ulcer, intestinal perforation due to CMV ulcers, pericardiotomy for tamponnade, etc. (DPK-personal observations).

Though the literature is unsettled, there is no compelling reason to avoid surgery simply based upon the presence of HIV infection, or of AIDS. However, prior to resorting to surgery, attempts should be made to improve the patient's status and maximize the chance of a successful outcome. This involves aggressive treatment of the local condition, including the patient's underlying medical complications, local infection, local inflammatory disease and nutritional status. Ultimately, the decision to operate and its timing rests with the consulting surgeon, who must weigh the expected risks and benefits of the surgical procedure, as well as the risks of not operating.

In conclusion, anorectal diseases are common and serious complications of AIDS. Their etiology is related directly to the effects of immune deficiency and, in many cases, to the presence of previously acquired traumatic and infectious diseases. An emerging body of clinical evidence indicates that effective suppressive and even curative treatments can be adminstered for many of the anorectal complications of AIDS. While the underlying disease state and immune deficiency may not be affected, the colorectal surgeon can play an important role in the treatment of a patient with AIDS.

Acknowledgement: This work was supported by grant no. 21414 from the National Institutes of Health.

References

1. Nossal GJV. Current Concepts; Immunology—The basic components of the immune system. *New Engl J Med* 1987; **316**:1320–5.
2. Hodges JR, Wright R. Normal immune responses in the gut and liver. *Clin Sci* 1982; **63**:339–47.
3. Guy-Grand D, Griscelli C, Vassalli P. The mouse gut lymphocyte, a novel type of

T cell: nature, origin and trafficking in normal and graft-vs-host conditions. *J Exp Med* 1978; **148**:1661–77.

4. Tomasi TB, Larson L, Challacombe S, McNabb P. Mucosal immunity: the origin and migration patterns of cells in the secretory system. *J Allergy Clin Immunol* 1980; **65**:12–19.

5. Kealy WF. Colonic lymphoid–glandular complex (microbursa): nature and morphology. *J Clin Pathol* 1976; **29**:241–4.

6. Wolf JL, Bye WA. The membraneous epithelial (M) cell and the mucosal immune system. *Ann Rev Med* 1984; **35**:95–112.

7. Janossy G, Tidman N, Selby WS, Thomas JA, Granger S. Human T lymphocytes of inducer and suppressor type occupy different micronenvironments. *Nature* 1980; **288**:81–4.

8. Selby WS, Janossy G, Goldstein G, Jewell DP. T lymphocyte subsets in human intestinal mucosa: the distribution and relationship to MHC-derived antigens. *Clin Exp Immunol* 1981; **44**:453–8.

9. Befus AD, Goodacre R, Dyce N, Bienenstock J. Mast cell heterogeneity in man. 1: Histologic studies of the intestine. *Int Arch Allergy App Immunol* 1985; **76**:232–6.

10. Hodges JR, Wright R. Normal immune responses in the gut and liver. *Clin Sci* 1982; **63**:339–47.

11. Green DR, Gold J, St Martin S, Gershon R, Gershon RK. Microenvironmental immunoregulation: possible role of contrasuppressor cells in maintaining immune responses in gut-associated lymphoid tissues. *Proc Natl Acad Sci USA* 1982; **79**:889–92.

12. Kagnoff MF. Oral tolerance. *Ann NY Acad Sci* 1982; **392**:248–264.

13. Edwards PAW. Is mucus a selective barrier for macromolecules? *Br Med Bull* 19; **34**:55–6.

14. Zubrzycki L, Spaulding EH. Studies on the stability of the normal fecal flora. *J Bacteriol* 1962; **83**:968–74.

15. Sakata T. Stimulatory effect of short chain fatty acids on epithelial cell proliferation in rat intestine: a possible explanation for trophic effects of fermentable fibre, gut microbes and luminal trophic factors. *Br J Nutr* 1987; **58**:95–108.

16. Bartlett JG, Chang T, Taylor NS, Onderdonk AB. Colitis induced by *Clostridium difficile*. *Rev Infect Dis* 1979; **1**:370–8.

17. Gottlieb MS, Schroff R, Schanker HM, *et al*. *Pneumocystis carinii* pneumonia and mucosal candidiasis in previously healthy homosexual men: evidence of a newly acquired cellular immunodeficiency. *N Engl J Med* 1981; **305**:1425–31.

18. Siegel FP, Lopez C, Hammer GS, *et al*. Severe acquired immunodeficiency in male homosexuals manifested by chronic perianal ulcerative herpes simplex lesions. *New Engl J Med* 1981; **305**:1439–44.

19. Berkelman RB, Heyward WL, Stehr-Green JK, Curran JW. Epidemiology of human immunodeficiency virus infection and acquired immunodeficiency syndrome. *Ann Intern Med* 1989; **86**:761–70.

20. Friedland GH, Saltzman BR, Rogers MR, *et al*. Lack of household transmission of HTLV-III. *New Engl J Med* 1986; **314**:344–9.

21. Friedland G, Kahl P, Saltzman B, *et al*. Additional evidence for lack of transmission of HIV infection by close interpersonal (casual) contact. *AIDS* 1990; **4**:639–44.

22. Barre-Sinoussi F, Chermann JC, Rey F, *et al*. Isolation of a T-lymphocytotropic retrovirus from a patient at risk for acquired immunodeficiency syndrome. *Science* 1983; **20**:868–71.

23. Gallo RC, Salahuhdin SZ, Popovic M, *et al*. Frequent detection and isolation of cytopathic retroviruses (HTLV-III) from patients with AIDS and at risk for AIDS. *Science* 1984; **224**:500–3.

24. Clavel F, Mansinho K, Chamaret S, *et al*. Human immunodeficiency virus type-2

infection associated with AIDS in West Africa. *New Engl J Med* 1987; **316**:1180–85.
25. Wong-Staal F, Gallo RC. Human T-lymphotropic retroviruses. *Nature* 1985; **317**:395–403.
26. Desrosiers RC, Letvin NL. Animal models for acquired immunodeficiency syndrome. *Rev Infect Dis* 1987; **9**:438–46.
27. Daigleish AG, Beverly PCL, Clapham PR, *et al*. The CD4 (T4) antigen is an essential component of the receptor for the AIDS virus. *Nature* 1984; **312**:763–7.
28. Gartner S, Markovits P, Markovitz DM, *et al*. The role of mononuclear phagocytes in HTLV-III/LAV infection. *Science* 1986; **233**:215–19.
29. Fox CF, Kotler D, Tierney A, *et al*. Detection of HIV-1 RNA in lamina propria of patients with AIDS and gastrointestinal disease. *J Infect Dis* 1989; **159**:467–71.
30. Nelson JA, Wiley CA, Reynolds-Kohler C, *et al*. Human immunodeficiency virus detected in bowel epithelium from patients with gastrointestinal symptoms. *Lancet* 1988; **2**:259–62.
31. Saag MS, Hahn BH, Gibbons J, *et al*. Extensive variation of human immunodeficiency virus type-1 *in vivo*. *Nature* 1988; **344**:440–4.
32. Koyanagi Y, Miles S, Mitsuyasu RT, Merrill JE, Vintners HV, Chen ISY. Dual infection of the central nervous system by AIDS viruses with distinct cellular tropisms. *Science* 1987; **236**:819–22.
33. Cann AJ, Karn J. Molecular biology of HIV: new insights into the virus life-cycle. *AIDS* 1989; **3**(Suppl. 1):S19–S34.
34. Rooke R, Tremblay M, Soudeyns H, *et al*. Isolation of drug-resistant variants of HIV-1 from patients on long-term zidovudine therapy. *AIDS* 1989; **3**:411–15.
35. Davis MG, Kenney SC, Kamine J, *et al*. Immediate–early gene region of human cytomegalovirus trans-activates the promoter of human immunodeficiency virus. *Proc Natl Acad Sci USA* 1987; **84**:8642–6.
36. Duh EJ, Maury WJ, Folks TM, Fauci AS, Rabson AB. Tumor necrosis factor A activates hyman immunodeficiency virus type-1 through induction of nuclear factor binding to the NF kappa B sites in the long terminal repeat. *Proc Natl Acad Sci USA* 1989; **86**:5874–8.
37. Tyler DS, Nastala CL, David Stanley S, *et al*. GP120 specific cellular cytotoxicity in HIV-1 seropositive individuals; evidence for circulating CD16+ effector cells armed *in vivo* with cytophilic antibody. *J Immunol* 1989; **142**:1177–82.
38. Reinherz EL, Schlossman SF. The differentiation and function of human T lymphocytes. *Cell* 1980; **19**:821–7.
39. Rodgers VD, Fassett R, Kagnoff MF. Abnormalities in intestinal mucosal T cells in homosexual populations including those with the lymphadenopathy syndrome and acquired immunodeficiency syndrome. *Gastroenterology* 1986; **90**:552–8.
40. Rook AH, Masur H, Lane HC, *et al*. Interleukin-2 enhances the depressed natural killer and cytomegalovirus-specific cytotoxic activities of lymphocytes from patients with the acquired immune deficiency syndrome. *J Clin Invest* 1983; **72**:398–403.
41. Kotler DP, Tierney AR, Scholes JV. Intestinal plasma cell alterations in the acquired immunodeficiency syndrome. *Dig Dis Sci* 1987; **32**:129–38.
42. Kotler DP, Wang J, Pierson R. Studies of body composition in patients with the Acquired Immunodeficiency Syndrome. *Am J Clin Nutr* 1985; **42**:1255–65.
43. Kotler DP, Tierney AR, Francisco A, Wang J, Pierson RN. The magnitude of body cell mass depletion determines the timing of death from wasting in AIDS. *Am J Clin Nutr* 1989; **50**:444–7.
44. Mullen JL, Gertner MH, Buzby GP, *et al*. Implications of malnutrition in the surgical patient. *Arch Surg* 1979; **114**:121–5.
45. Kotler DP, Tierney AR, Ferraro R, Cuff P, Wang J, Pierson RN, Heymsfield S. Effect of enteral feeding upon body cell mass in AIDS. *Am J Clin Nutr* (in press).

46. Kotler DP, Tierney AR, Wang J, Pierson RN. Effect of home total parenteral nutrition upon body composition in AIDS. *J Parenter Enteral Nutr* (in press).
47. Von Roenn JH, Murphy RL, Weber KM, Williams LM, Weitzman SA. Megesterol acetate for treatment of cachexia associated with human immunodeficiency virus infection. *Ann Intern Med* 1988; **109**:840–1.
48. Kotler DP, Tierney AR, Altilio D, Wang J, Pierson RN. Body mass repletion during ganciclovir therapy of cytokmegalovirus infections in patients with the acquired immunodeficiency syndrome. *Arch Int Med* 1989; **149**:901–5.
49. Scannell KA. Surgery and human immunodeficiency virus disease. *J Acq Immunodef Virus Synd* 1989; **2**:43–53.
50. Robinson G, Wilson SE, Williams RA. Surgery in patients with acquired immunodeficiency syndrome. *Arch Surg* 1987; **122**:170–5.
51. Wexner SD, Smithy WB, Milsom JW, Dailey TH. The surgical management of anorectal diseases in AIDS and pre-AIDS patients. *Dis Col Rectum* 1986; **29**:719–23.
52. Schneider PA, Abrams DI, Rayner AA, Hohn DC. Immunodeficiency associated thrombocytopenic purpura. *Arch Surg* 1987; **122**:1175–8.

2

Epidemiology of HIV transmission by anoreceptive intercourse
Steven D Wexner

Introduction

The human immunodeficiency virus (HIV) is a sexually transmitted retro-virus that infects and can progressively destroy the population of helper–inducer lymphocytes. This helper cell population is known as either OKT4, CD4 or T4 lymphocytes, synonymous terms referring to the surface epitopes [1]. The HIV may also infect monocytes, macrophages and other cells [2]. It is self-evident that compromise of the OKT4, monocyte and macrophage populations can have a disastrous effect on the patient's immune system. This supposition is certainly proven when one considers the plethora of manifestations of HIV. These maladies range from subclinical laboratory abnormalities to the full-blown spectrum of the acquired immune deficiency syndrome. This chapter will review that portion of the epidemiology of HIV infection which is germane to the population of HIV-infected patients who develop anorectal disorders.

Prevalence

Up to February 1990, more than 123 000 cases of AIDS had been diagnosed in the USA [3]. In addition an estimated 1 000 000 to 2 000 000 people in the USA were believed to be infected with AIDS [4]. It is expected that between 25% and 35% of those infected with HIV will develop AIDS within two years of infection [4]. Thus a conservative estimate is that by the year 1991, 250 000 Americans will carry the diagnosis of AIDS [5]. Based upon well-established trends, in the absence of discovery of a cure or prevention for AIDS, the mortality rate for this group will be close to 100% [6]. Fig. 2.1 shows the prevalence rate for AIDS in the USA in 1989, and Fig. 2.2 shows the continued increase in its incidence.

Population at risk

Table 2.1 shows the risk factors in the male and female populations. Male AIDS patients outnumber females by a factor of 10, and 75% of males are

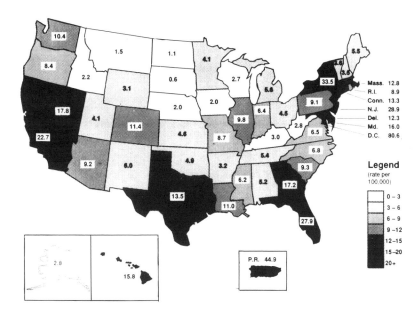

Figure 2.1 AIDS annual rates per 100 000 population in the USA, for cases reported in 1989. Reprinted with permission from reference 3.

homosexual or bisexual. The significance of these facts will be discussed in this chapter.

The single most common risk factor for infection with HIV or for the subsequent development of AIDS is homosexuality. This pattern of HIV transmission accounts for 68% of all cases of AIDS in the adult and

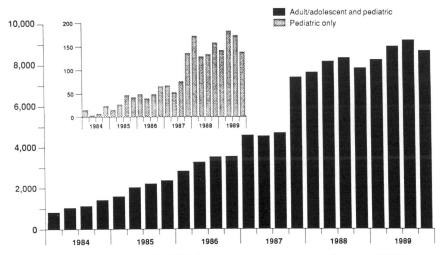

Figure 2.2 AIDS cases in the USA by quarter year, reported January 1984 to December 1989. Reprinted with permission from reference 3.

Table 2.1 Adult/adolescent AIDS cases in the USA, by sex, exposure category, and race/ethnicity, reported up to the end of 1989

Male exposure category	White, not Hispanic	Black, not Hispanic	Hispanic	Asian/ Pacific Islander	American Indian/ Alaskan Native	Totals§
	No. (%)	No. (%)	No. (%)	No. (%)	No. (%)	No. (%)
Male homosexual/bisexual contact	50 447 (80)	11 501 (45)	7 386 (47)	533 (81)	79 (62)	70 093 (67)
Intravenous (IV) drug use (heterosexual)	3 734 (6)	8 914 (35)	5 989 (38)	17 (3)	12 (9)	18 721 (18)
Male homosexual/bisexual contact and IV drug use	4 794 (8)	2 118 (8)	1 162 (7)	12 (2)	21 (16)	8 117 (8)
Hemophilia/coagulation disorder	862 (1)	68 (0)	79 (1)	15 (2)	6 (5)	1 034 (1)
Heterosexual contact:	353 (1)	1 773 (7)	172 (1)	5 (1)	1 (1)	2 308 (2)
Sex with IV drug user	*232*	*463*	*119*	*1*	*1*	*816*
Sex with person with hemophilia	*3*	*1*	*–*	*–*	*–*	*4*
Born in Pattern-II* country	*2*	*1 178*	*7*	*3*	*–*	*1 193*
Sex with person born in Pattern-II country	*23*	*24*	*2*	*–*	*–*	*49*
Sex with transfusion recipient with HIV infection	*14*	*6*	*1*	*–*	*–*	*22*
Sex with HIV-infected person, risk not specified	*79*	*101*	*43*	*1*	*–*	*224*
Receipt of blood transfusion, blood components, or tissue†	1 341 (2)	239 (1)	148 (1)	34 (5)	1 (1)	1 768 (2)
Other/undetermined‡	1 224 (2)	1 097 (4)	738 (5)	39 (6)	8 (6)	3 134 (3)
Male subtotal	62 755(100)	25 710(100)	15 674(100)	655(100)	128(100)	105 175(100)
Female exposure category						
IV drug use	1 175 (41)	3 171 (58)	1 110 (52)	11 (18)	14 (56)	5 491 (52)
Hemophilia/coagulation disorder	24 (1)	3 (0)	1 (0)	–	–	28 (0)
Heterosexual contact:	782 (27)	1 730 (32)	771 (36)	22 (36)	8 (32)	3 322 (31)
Sex with IV drug user	*402*	*991*	*643*	*10*	*3*	*2 055*
Sex with bisexual male	*183*	*117*	*46*	*5*	*1*	*353*
Sex with person with hemophilia	*44*	*2*	*1*	*1*	*–*	*48*
Born in Pattern-II country	*1*	*433*	*2*	*1*	*–*	*439*
Sex with person born in Pattern-II country	*1*	*32*	*–*	*–*	*–*	*33*
Sex with transfusion recipient with HIV infection	*47*	*4*	*7*	*1*	*–*	*59*
Sex with HIV-infected person, risk not specified	*104*	*151*	*72*	*4*	*4*	*335*
Receipt of blood transfusion, blood components, or tissue	709 (25)	210 (4)	118 (6)	22 (36)	2 (8)	1 062 (10)
Other/undetermined	200 (7)	374 (7)	119 (6)	6 (10)	1 (4)	708 (7)
Female subtotal	2 890(100)	5 488(100)	2 119(100)	61(100)	25(100)	10 611(100)
Total	65 645	31 198	17 793	716	153	115 786

*MMWR 1988; 37:286–8, 293–5.
†Includes six transfusion recipients who received blood screened for HIV antibody, and one tissue recipient.
‡'Other' refers to two health-care workers who seroconverted to HIV and developed AIDS after occupational exposure to HIV-infected blood. 'Undetermined' refers to patients whose mode of exposure to HIV was unknown. This includes patients under investigation; patients who died, were lost to follow-up, or refused interview; and patients whose mode of exposure to HIV remained undetermined after investigation.
§Includes 253 males and 28 females whose race/ethnicity is unknown.
Source: Reprinted with permission from reference 3.

adolescent populations reported up to December 1989 [3]. The mode of transmission weighs heavily upon the subsequent manifestations, as the homosexual and bisexual male populations tend to present with a different spectrum of disorders than do those HIV-infected persons who are hetero-sexual, intravenous drug abusers, or hemophiliacs [7].

In a study by Wexner and coworkers it was found that 15% of patients with AIDS or what was formerly known as AIDS-related complex (ARC) and pre-AIDS presented with anorectal pathology prior to the diagnosis of AIDS [8]. In addition, 116 of 340 AIDS, ARC and pre-AIDS patients (34%) manifested some form of anorectal disease during their illness. The single most common anorectal manifestation was perianal sepsis, observed in 58% of the patients. Other commonly noted diseases included perianal con-dylomata acuminata, Kaposi's sarcoma, cytomegalovirus, carcinoma-in-situ, lymphoma, tuberculous proctitis, perianal histoplasmoma, invasive carcinoma and non-healing anal ulcers. Perianal herpes simplex virus infections were notably absent from this series because only those patients who underwent surgery for their anorectal conditions were reported. Other authors have reported similar findings [9–11].

Risk factors for transmission

Rietmeijer and associates performed a multivariate analysis of homosexual men to determine which risk factors were significant for the development of AIDS [12]. They found that the number of episodes of receptive anal intercourse, the age at which such intercourse started, the use of erotic enemas, sexual contact with an AIDS or ARC partner, and a history of hepatitis B, were all independently associated with HIV infection. Other studies have shown that increasing the frequency of anal receptive inter-course (ARI) and the number of partners both correlate directly with the prevalence of HIV seropositivity [13–15]. Chmiel and colleagues have added to this list of significant factors receptive 'fisting', anorectal gonorrhea, syphilis or herpes, and elevated cytomegalovirus (CMV) antibody titers [16]. Although multiple studies have reported that receptive 'fisting' is an independent risk factor for the development of AIDS, it is difficult to prove this. The difficulty lies in the fact that most homosexual and bisexual men also practice either ARI, oroanal intercourse, or both.

Simonsen and coworkers reported that uncircumcised men and those with a history of genital ulceration were at higher risk for the development of HIV diseases [17]. A subsequent report by the same group assessed HIV seropositivity in a group of 422 men who had sexually transmitted diseases (STDs) acquired from female prostitutes [18]. Logistic regression analysis showed that increased risk of seroconversion was independently associated with being uncircumcised, with genital ulceration, and with regular contact with prostitutes. These sexual practices which have been repeatedly associ-ated with an increased risk of HIV infection are listed in Table 2.2.

Although anal receptive intercourse is probably the single most common method of HIV transmission, orogenital intercourse has also been reported to be associated with seroconversion [19]. Thus in order to reduce the risk of

Table 2.2   Sexual practices associated with increased risk of infection with HIV

Highest risk factors*
   Contact with infected semen or blood
      Receptive anal intercourse (especially with ejaculation)
      Receptive vaginal intercourse (especially with ejaculation)
      Fellatio involving contact with semen

Moderate/significant risk factors*
   Insertive anal intercourse
   Insertive vaginal intercourse
   Brachioproctic eroticism
   Use of enemas/rectal douches
   Use of sexual devices
   Oral–anal contact
   Fellatio without contact with semen

Lesser risk factors†
   Contact with urine
   Mutual masturbation with ejaculation on partner
   'Deep' kissing
   Cunnilingus

*Based on current epidemiologic evidence.
†Based on weaker evidence and/or presumed risk.
Source: Adapted from Glasel M, High-risk sexual practices in the transmission of AIDS. In reference 7: 355–67.

HIV seroconversion, the penis should be covered with a condom. As added protection, nonoxynol-9 should be used as well [20]. Nonoxynol-9 has been shown to be not only spermicidal, but also to inhibit *in vitro* growth of *Treponema pallidum*, *Neisseria gonorrheaoeae*, *Chlamydia trachomatis*, herpes simplex virus, and HIV [20].

Sexual intercourse with female prostitutes is certainly an important vehicle of transmission of HIV. Khabbaz and associates tested 1305 female prostitutes from eight geographic areas of the USA [21]. Overall, 6.7% were HIV seropositive with seroprevalence rates ranging from 0% in Southern Nevada to 25.4% in Newark, New Jersey. Seropositivity for HIV was independently associated with hepatitis B seropositivity, intravenous drug use, race and number of years of sexual activity.

Overall, approximately 4% of all AIDS cases in the USA have been attributed to heterosexual contact with a person at risk for HIV infection [22]. Nearly 40% of these seropositive heterosexual AIDS patients had histories of sexually transmitted disease. Despite the fact that heterosexual transmission of HIV has been documented after a single heterosexual contact, there are other cases in which no evidence of transmission exists after hundreds of contacts with an infected person [23].

Sexual transmission from male to female is thought to be more efficient than transmission from female to male; genital ulcer disease probably increases the risk of acquiring HIV infection [22]. The incidence of heterosexual spread of AIDS is greater in blacks than in whites in the USA [3]. This may be explained either by the larger proportion of bisexual men among black homosexuals, or a greater overlap between bisexual and intravenous drug using black men than among their white counterparts [24]. Alternatively, this discrepancy might reflect an earlier introduction of HIV into the black heterosexual population [24].

Sexual promiscuity, as in the homosexual population, appears to be a risk factor for HIV transmission in the heterosexual population [25]. Masters and coworkers compared the HIV-antibody status of 400 heterosexuals (200 men and 200 women) who reported six or more sexual partners per year with the antibody status of 400 heterosexuals (200 men and 200 women) who maintained monogamy for five years [25]. All of these patients were allegedly carefully screened for, and did not have, any risk factors for AIDS. Seven per cent of the women and 5% of the 'promiscuous' men were HIV seropositive, whereas only one man who practiced monogamy was seropositive (0.05%).

Despite the slight increase in heterosexual spread seen over the last few years, there exist far fewer heterosexual than homosexual men with AIDS [3]. Several possible explanations for this phenomenon have been posed. First, the mean number of sexual partners is greater in the latter group. In early studies conducted by the Centers for Disease Control (CDC), homosexual AIDS patients had a median of 1116 lifetime sexual partners [26]. This was substantially different from the median of 40 reported for male heterosexual intravenous drug users with AIDS. In simple mathematical terms, as the number of partners increases, so too does the probability of exposure to an infected partner [27]. The second reason is that the reservoir of HIV is much greater in the homosexual male than in either the male or female heterosexual populations. Again, mathematics predict that for each random, anonymous sexual encounter, a homosexual male is more likely to infect his partner than is his heterosexual counterpart [24]. In addition, anal receptive intercourse may be more efficient in the transmission of HIV than is vaginal intercourse [28]. Perhaps the columnar epithelium which comprises the rectum and upper anal canal is more easily lacerated than is the stout stratified squamous epithelium of the vagina. Anal-receptive intercourse has been identified as an independent predictor of HIV seropositivity in women as well as in men [7]. The likelihood of HIV seroconversion in women who practice ARI is approximately twice that of those who limit their behavior to oral or vaginal intercourse. Kingsley and coworkers showed that ARI was responsible for nearly all HIV seroconversions in a group of 2507 homosexual men prospectively followed for six months [29]. Lastly, there may be cofactors which enhance or facilitate HIV transmission among homosexual men. These sexually transmitted diseases may include herpes simplex virus, cytomegalovirus, hepatitis B, gonorrhea, syphilis, or the human papilloma virus. As has been previously mentioned, genital ulceration is an independent prognosticator for HIV seroconversion [16,18].

Recent data have suggested that Kaposi's sarcoma is a sexually transmitted disease. Beral and associates from the Center for Disease Control reported that KS is 20 000 times more common in AIDS patients than in the general population [30]. Although this may seem self-evident, they also noted that KS was 300-fold more common in AIDS patients than in patients whose immunocompromise was due to other etiologies. The most interesting revelation in their study, however, was that KS was 21-fold more common in homosexual or bisexual male AIDS patients than in male hemophiliacs with AIDS. The risk was greatest in homosexual and bisexual men in New York and California. This difference between the homosexual/ bisexual and the heterosexual male population may be even more profound, as the authors suspect bias towards misclassification of homosexual or bisexual men into other risk groups. Interestingly, among women with heterosexually acquired HIV, those whose partners were bisexual men had a fourfold increase in prevalence of KS over those with other sexual partners.

Apparently Kaposi's sarcoma can occur in the homosexual and bisexual male population even in the absence of HIV infection [31]. Friedman-Kien and colleagues reported six cases of HIV-negative homosexual or bisexual men from New York with KS. These data raise two considerations. First, KS may be a sexually transmitted disease acquired independently of HIV infection. Second, the agent responsible for KS may not be the HIV but a second infectious agent. However, the two infectious agents may be simultaneously transmitted and synergistic. Clearly, however, anal receptive intercourse has adverse sequelae over and above HIV seroconversion.

Anal receptive intercourse as a risk factor

In order to understand the currently favored hypothesis regarding the role of ARI in HIV seroconversion, it is important to review a sequence of discoveries. First, antisperm antibodies were detected in the serum of some homosexual males; these antibodies cross-reacted with certain T-lympho-cyte surface antigens [32]. Based on this fact, Sonnabend and associates felt that exposure to allogenic sperm may play an important etiologic role in the development of impaired T-cell immunoregulation in male homosexuals [34]. Mavligit and colleagues prospectively evaluated 30 asymptomatic monogamously paired homosexual males. Evidence for allogenic immuniz-ation existed among 19 of 26 homosexual males who were the recipients during ARI. No evidence for any form of alloimmunization, however, was found in four males who were exclusively sperm 'donors'. In this study, immune dysregulation was in the form of a reduced effector/suppresor T-cell ratio (less than 1.0), seen exclusively in ARI recipients, and a subnor-mal local graft versus host reaction. Similar evidence for alloimmunization was associated with a reversed T-helper cell subset population in the female patient who routinely practiced ARI, resulting in a high frequency of allogenic immunization and leading possibly to the development of AIDS.

This theory is a tenable one in light of the topography of the anorectum and the other factors discussed in the last section. Most importantly, perhaps, the single layer of columnar epithelium lining the rectum not only permits laceration and abrasion more readily than does the vaginal lining, but also is richly vascularized and thus predisposed to transmucosal antigen absorption. The intense immunogenicity of sperm, compounded, perhaps, in a synergistic fashion with the rectal flora, may generate chronic antigenic stimulation. This is analogous to the transanal transmission of hepatitis B.

The fact that colorectal epithelial cells are receptive to the HIV was initially demonstrated by Adachi and coworkers [35]. In this study cultured colo-rectal cells were found to be susceptible to direct infection with HIV. The first clinical correlation with this finding was reported by Nelson and associates [36]. The authors evaluated 13 HIV-infected patients with a history of chronic diarrhea of unknown etiology and one HIV-seropositive patient with no gastrointestinal complaints. The protocol called for colorectal and duodenal biopsy followed by *in situ* hybridization. Using this technique, viral nucleic acid was detected in 7 out of 11 patients' rectal biopsy specimens. None of 12 bowel biopsy specimens from seronegative individuals showed hybridization. The rectum was the area of bowel which showed the highest number of HIV-infected cells. In most cases, HIV nucleic acid was detected primarily at the bases of the crypts. This study was extremely important in proving that colorectal mucosa can be infected by HIV. The presence of such susceptible cells in an area prone to trauma and subsequent insemination could be at least partly responsible for the known risk of infection for receptive partners during ARI.

Diagnosis

There are, at present, three methods of diagnosis of HIV infection. The first method entails isolation of the virus through cell culture. This technique requires identification of reverse-transcriptase activity. Secondly, HIV-specific nucleic acid sequences may be observed in cells. Lastly, either HIV-specific antigens or antibodies may be found in body fluids. The most widely tested, widely available, and therefore widely accepted of the groups of assays are those which identify HIV antibodies. Certainly HIV testing is of paramount importance in the diagnosis of AIDS.

The diagnosis of AIDS is now affixed only to persons who have at least one well-defined life-threatening clinical problem that is clearly a result of HIV-induced immunosuppression. The CDC surveillance definition of AIDS was revised in 1987 [37]. The presence of *Pneumocystis carinii* pneumonia, other life-threatening opportunisitc infections, or Kaposi's sarcoma continue to define most cases of AIDS in the USA. The diagnosis of AIDS does not require HIV seropositivity but does require the fulfillment of the criteria outlined in Table 2.3. Basically, using the redefined CDC terminology, patients are labeled as having AIDS if they have serologic evidence of HIV infection and one or more other immunodeficiency-associated maladies. These include B-cell non-Hodgkin's lymphomas, HIV dementia, HIV wasting, and tuberculosis.

Although the CDC surveillance definitions are useful in the western world, not all developing countries have access to the HIV-antibody assays. For this reason, the World Health Organization (WHO) has developed a provisional clinical case definition of AIDS for purposes of surveillance (Table 2.4). These clinically defined cases of AIDS include patients with disseminated Kaposi's sarcoma, cryptococcal meningitis, or a combination of major and minor signs and symptoms of HIV infection. The signs which are germane to the coloproctologist include chronic unexplained diarrhea, chronic and progressive mucocutaneous herpes simplex virus, and a history of herpes zoster virus within the previous five years.

Table 2.3   AIDS—Revised surveillance definition of the Centers for Disease Control (CDC)

HIV status positive, negative* or unknown†
One or more of the following diagnoses proven by microscopy or culture:
  Pneumocytis carinii pneumonia
  Candidiasis of the esophagus, trachea, bronchi, or lungs
  Extrapulmonary *Mycobacterium avium* complex or *M. kansasii* infection
  Herpes simplex virus infection causing bronchitis, pneumonitis or esophagitis,
    or a mucocutaneous ulcer persisting >1 month‡
  Cytomegalovirus infection of an internal organ other than liver‡
  Toxoplasmosis of an internal organ‡
  Cryptosporidiosis with diarrhea persisting >1 month
  Extraintestinal strongyloidiasis
  Progressive multifocal leukoencephalopathy
  Kaposi's sarcoma (<60 years of age)
  Primary lymphoma of the brain (<60 years of age)
  Pulmonary lymphoid hyperplasia or lymphoid interstitial pneumonitis
    (<13 years of age)

HIV status positive
One or more of the following diagnoses proven by microscopy or culture:
  Kaposi's sarcoma (at any age)
  Primary lymphoma of the brain (at any age)
  B-cell non-Hodgkin's lymphomas of the small non-cleaved (Burkitt-like) or
    immunoblastic sarcoma (large cell lymphoma, diffuse histiocytic or
    undifferentiated lymphoma, reticulum cell sarcoma, or high-grade
    lymphoma) types
  HIV dementia complex
  HIV wasting syndrome (enteropathic AIDS, 'slim' disease)
  Extrapulmonary or disseminated tuberculosis or other non-cutaneous
    mycobacterial infection other than leprosy
  Extrapulmonary or disseminated histoplasmosis
  Extrapulmonary or disseminated coccidioidomycosis
  Isopsoriasis with diarrhea persisting >1 month
  Nocardiosis
  Salmonella septicemia
  Two or more bacterial infections within 2 years of the following types in a child
    <13 years of age not predisposed by chronic lung disease: septicemia,
    pneumonia, meningitis, or brain abscess caused by *Legionella*, *Hemophilus*,
    Streptococcus (including pneumococcus), or another pyogenic bacterium

One or more or the following diagnoses not proven by microscopy or culture:
  Pneumocytis carinii pneumonia
  Toxoplasmosis of an internal organ§
  Esophageal candidiasis
  Extrapulmonary or disseminated mycobacterial infection (acid-fast bacilli of
    undetermined species)
Progressive multifocal leukoencephalopathy
  Kaposi's sarcoma
  Pulmonary lymphoid hyperplasia or lymphoid interstitial pneumonitis
    (<13 years of age)

---

* AIDS is not excluded by negative HIV serology in patients with *Pneumocystis carinii* pneumonia or a T4 (T-helper) lymphocyte count <400/ml, since in some patients with

Table 2.4   AIDS—Provisional clinical surveillance definition of the World Health Organization

AIDS is defined as:*

Disseminated Kaposi's sarcoma
   or
Cryptococcal meningitis
   or

At least two major signs:	Plus at least one minor sign:
Weight loss >10%	Cough >1 month†
Diarrhea >1 month	General lymphadenopathy†
Fever >1 month	General pruritic dermatitis
	History of herpes zoster within 5 years
	Oropharyngeal candidiasis
	Chronic and progressive herpes simplex

*Excluding patients with other known causes of immunosuppression.
†Excluding patients with proven tuberculosis.
Source: Adapted from reference 38.

AIDS throughout the world

In Central and South America, Brazil clearly leads the list of AIDS cases reported. Despite the fact that over 2000 cases of AIDS have been identified, the per capita rates are lower in Brazil than they are in the Caribbean. The countries with the highest per capita rates of AIDS are Haiti, Trinidad, and Tobago. The most prevalent risk factor in Brazil is homosexuality, where-as in the Caribbean the type II pattern (heterosexual transmissions) predominates [7].

In Africa, heterosexual transmission is more common than in the USA, and the symptomatology of the disease is varied. In Africa, HIV enteropathy (diarrhea-wasting syndrome; 'slim disease') is much more frequently observed than it is in the USA [39]. The presumptive diagnosis of AIDS is also confounded by the fact that several manifestations of AIDS, such as tuberculosis and KS, are endemic in Africa [7]. Therefore the HIV serology is of paramount importance in differentiation of the endemic from the much more highly aggressive epidemic variety. Migratory patterns have made AIDS, as in the West, largely an urban disease.

advanced immune deficiency hypogammaglobulinemia may supervene with reversion to HIV-antibody negative.
†If HIV status is unknown or negative, the following causes of immunodeficiency must be excluded: systemic corticosteroid, immunosuppressive, or cytotoxic therapy within 3 months; Hodgkin's disease, non-Hodgkin's lymphoma (other than brain lymphoma), lymphocytic leukemia, multiple myeloma, or other cancer of lymphoreticular or histiocytic tissue, or angioimmunoblastic lymphadenopathy within 3 months; any genetic, congenital, or acquired immunodeficiency syndrome atypical of HIV infection.
‡Over 1 month of age.
Source: Adapted from reference 37.

Staging systems

The simplest quantifier of immune function of HIV-infected patients is the CD4+ cell count. However, data on the helper–inducer/suppressor ratios are not always readily available in the clinical setting. The CDC has devised a clinical staging system for HIV infection which is exceedingly useful (Table 2.45) [40]. Despite the elegant simplicity of this staging system, its prognostic value has yet to be ascertained. An alternative staging system is the one proposed by the Walter Reed Group (Table 2.5) [41]. Unfortunately this latter system is even more cumbersome than that proposed by the CDC, as it necessitates knowledge of HIV status, D4+ cell count, cutaneous energy status, and presence or absence of opportunistic infections and lymphadenopathy. This combined clinical and laboratory staging system is of theoretical value as it is an accurate barometer of the patient's immune

Table 2.5   Staging systems for conditions related to HIV

Centers for Disease Control (CDC) classification system

Group	Description
I	Acute infection
II	Asymptomatic infection
III	Persistent generalized lymphadenopathy
IV	Other disease
Subgroup A	Constitutional disease
Subgroup B	Neurologic disease
Subgroup C	Secondary infectious diseases
Category C-1	Specified secondary infectious diseases listed in the CDC surveillance definition for AIDS[†]
Category C-2	Other specified secondary infectious diseases
Subgroup D	Secondary cancers, including those within the CDC surveillance definition for AIDS[†]
Subgroup E	Other conditions

Walter Reed classification system

Stage	HIV antibody or culture	Chronic lymphaden-opathy	CD4+ cell count/ml	Cutaneous Anergy	Thrush	Oppor-tunistic infection
WR0	−	−	>400	None	−	−
WR1	+*	−	>400	None	−	−
WR2	+*	+*	>400	None	−	−
WR3	+*	+/−	<400*	None	−	−
WR4	+*	+/−	<400*	Partial*	−	−
WR5	+*	+/−	<400	Complete or partial	+*	−
WR6	+*	+/−	<400	Complete or partial	+/−	+*

*Indicates critical features of each Walter Reed (WR) stage.
[†]See Table 2.3 for the CDC surveillance definition for AIDS.
Sources: References 40 and 41.

status. The Walter Reed staging system, for these reasons, probably has a better relationship to both pathobiology and prognosis than does the CDC system.

Conclusions

It is not the aim of this chapter to provide a definitive treatise on the global epidemiology of AIDS. However, it is of paramount importance that the colorectal surgeon be familiar with these epidemiologic associations of AIDS relative to the colorectum. Those patients whose HIV infection is acquired in a type II (heterosexual) pattern are far less likely to present with colorectal manifestations of AIDS than are homosexual and bisexual men [42]. In 15–30% of cases of AIDS, the initial diagnostic manouvers are prompted by patient presentation with colorectal pathology [8,43–45]. These manifestations range from the obvious lesions such as Kaposi's sarcoma and condylomata acuminata to the more protean, including non-healing anal 'fissures' and perianal lymphoma. Although treatment of the AIDS patient with colorectal pathology is difficult enough, diagnosis of AIDS or of HIV infection is even more challenging. In order to practice colorectal surgery in the 1990s one must be fully cognizant not only of the clinical colorectal manifestations of HIV infection, but also of the risk factors and transmission patterns of the disease.

References

1. Popovic M, Sargadharan MG, Read E, *et al*. Detection, isolation, and continuous production or cytopathic retrovirus (HTLV-III) from patients from AIDS and pre-AIDS. *Science* 1984; **225**:491–506.
2. Gartner S, Markovits P, Markovitz DM, *et al*. The role of mononuclear phagocytes in HYLV-III/LAW infection. *Science* 1986; **233**:215–20.
3. Centers for Disease Control. HIV/AIDS Surveillance Report, February 1990: 1–22.
4. Curran JW, Jaffe WH, Hady AM, *et al*. Epidemiology of HIV infection and AIDS in the United States. *Science* 1988, **239**:610–18.
5. Coolfont report: A public health service plan for prevention and control of AIDS and AIDS virus. *Public Health Service Report* 1986; **101**:341–8.
6. Lui KJ, Darrow WW, Rutherford GW. A model-based estimate of the mean incubation period for AIDS in homosexual men. *Science* 1988; **240**:1333–5.
7. DeVita VT, Hellman S, Rosenberg SA (eds). *AIDS: Etiology, Diagnosis, Treatment and Presentation* 92nd edn). Philadelphia: Lippincott, 1988.
8. Wexner SD, Smithy WB, Milsom JW, Dailey TH. The surgical management of anorectal diseses in AIDS and pre-AIDS patients. *Dis Col Rectum* 1986; **29**:719–23.
9. Kaplan LD. AIDS-associated lymphomas. *Infect Dis Clin N Am* 1988; **2**:525–32.
10. Croxson T, Chabon AB, Rorat E, Barash IM. Intraepithelial carcinoma of the anus in homosexual men. *Dis Col Rectum* 1984; **27**:325–30.
11. Wexner SD, Smithy WB, Trillo C, Hopkins BS, Dailey TH. Emergency colectomy for cytomegalovirus ileocolitis in patients with the acquired immune deficiency syndrome. *Dis Col Rectum* 1988; **31**:755–61.
12. Rietmeijer CAM, Penley KA, Cohn DL, Davidson AJ, Horsburgh CR, Judson

FN. Factors influencing the risk of infection with human immunodeficiency virus in homosexual men, Denver 1982–1985. *Sex Trans Dis* 1984; **16**:95–102.

13. Winkelstein W, Lyman DM, Padian N, *et al.* Sexual practices and risk of infection by the human immunodeficiency virus: the San Francisco Men's Health Study. *JAMA* 1987; **257**:321–5.

14. Darrow WW, Echenberg DF, Jaffe HW, *et al.* Risk factors for human immuno-deficiency virus (HIV) infections in homosexual men. *Am J Pub Health* 1987; **77**:479–83.

15. Moss AR, Osmond D, Bacchetti P, *et al.* Risk factors for AIDS and HIV seropositivity in homosexual men. *Am J Epidemiol* 1987; **125**:1035–47.

16. Chmiel JS, Detels R, Kaslow RA, *et al.* Factors associated with prevalent human immunodeficiency virus (HIV) infections in the multicenter AIDS cohort study. *Am J Epidemiol* 1987; **127**:568–77.

17. Simonson JN, Cameron DW, Gakinya MN, *et al.* Human immunodeficiency virus infection among men with sexually transmitted diseases. *New Engl J Med* 1988; **19**:274–8.

18. Cameron DW, Simonsen JN, D'Costa LJ, *et al.* Female to male transmission of human immunodeficiency virus type-1: risk factors for seroconversion in men. *Lancet* 1989; **1**(8660):402–7.

19. Goldberg DJ, Green St, Kennedy DH, Emslie JAN, Black JD. HIV and orogenital transmission (letter). *Lancet* 1988; **2**:1363.

20. Rietmeijer CAM, Krebs JW, Feorino PM, Judson FN. Condoms as physical and chemical barriers against human immunodeficiency virus. *JAMA* 1989; **250**:1851–3.

21. Khabbaz RF, Darrow WW, Hartley JM, *et al.* Seroprevalence and risk factors for HTLV-I/II infection among female prostitutes in the United States *JAMA* 1990; **2623**:60–4.

22. Berkelman RL, Heyward WL, Stehr-Green JK, Curran J. Epidemiology of human immunodeficiency virus infection and acquired immunodeficiency syndrome. *Am J Med* 1989; **86**:761–70.

23. Peterman TA, Stoneburner RL, Allen JR, *et al.* Risk of human immunodeficiency virus transmission from heterosexual adults with transfusion-associated infec-tions. *JAMA* 1988; **259**:55–8.

24. Haverkos HW, Edelman R. The epidemiology of acquired immunodeficiency syndrome among heterosexuals. *JAMA* 1988; **260**:1922–9.

25. Masters WH, Johnson VE, Kolodny RC. *Crisis: Heterosexual Behavior in the Age of AIDS.* New York: Grove Press, 1988: 47–68.

26. Guinan ME, Thomas PA, Pinsky PE, *et al.* Heterosexual and homosexual patients with the acquired immunodeficiency syndrome: a comparison of sur-veillance, interview, and laboratory data. *Ann Intern Med* 1984; **100**:213–8.

27. Padian N, Marquis L, Francis DP, *et al.* Male-to-female transmission of human immunodeficiency virus. *JAMA* 1987; **258**: 788–90.

28. Nicholson JKA, McDougal JS, Jaffe HW, *et al.* Exposure to human T-lympho-tropic virus type III/lymphodenopathy-associated virus, and immunologic ab-normalities in asymptomatic homosexual men. *Ann Intern Med* 1985; **103**:37–42.

29. Kinglsey LA, Detels R, Kaslow R, *et al.* Risk factors for seroconversion to human immunodeficiency virus among male homosexuals. *Lancet* 1987; **1**:345–9.

30. Beral V, Peterman TA, Berkelman RL, Jaffe HW. Kaposi's sarcoma among persons with AIDS or sexually transmitted infection. *Lancet* 1990; **335**:123–8.

31. Friedan-Kien AF, Saltzman BR, Cao Y, Mirabile M, Li JJ, Peterman TA. Kaposi's sarcoma in HIV-negative homosexual men. *Lancet* 1990; **335**:168–9.

32. Witkin SS, Sonnabend J. Immune responses to spermatazoa in homosexual men. *Fertil Steril* 1983; **39**:337–42.

33. Sonnabend J. Witkin SS, Pertilo DT. Acquired immunodeficiency syndrome,

opportunistic infections, and malignancies in male homosexuals: a hypothesis of etiologic factors in pathogenesis. *JAMA* 1983; **249**:2370–4.

34. Mavligit GM, Talpaz M, Hsia FT, *et al*. Chronic immune stimulation by sperm alloantigens. *JAMA* 1984; **251**:237–41.
35. Adachi A, Koenig S, Gendelman HE, *et al*. Productive, persistent infection of human colorectal cell lines with human immunodeficiency virus. *J Virol* 1987; **61**:209–13.
36. Nelson JA, Wiley CA, Reynolds-Kohler C, Reese CE, Martaretten W, Levy JA. Human immunodeficiency virus detected in bowel epithelium from patients with gastrointestinal symptoms. *Lancet* 1988; **2**: 259–62.
37. Centers for Disease Control. Revision of the CDC surveillance definition for acquired immunodeficiency syndrome. *MMWR* (Suppl.) 1987; **36**:1s–15s.
38. Colebunder R, Mann JM, Francis H, *et al*. Evaluation of a clinical case definition of acquired immunodeficiency syndrome in Africa. *Lancet* 1987; **1**: 492.
39. Serwadda D, Mugerwa RD, Serwankambo NK, *et al*. Slim disease: a new disease in Uganda and its association with HTLV-III infection. *Lancet* 1085; **2**: 849–50.
40. Centers for Disease Control. Classification system for human T-lymphotropic virus type III/lymphadenopathy-associated virus infections. *MMWR* 1986; **35**:334–41.
41. Redfield RR, Wright DC, Tramont EC. The Walter Reed staging classification for HTLV-III/LAV infection, *New Engl J Med* 1986; **317**:131–6.
42. Centers for Disease Control. Update: acquired immunodeficiency syndrome (AIDS)—worldwide. *MMWR* 1988; **37**:286–8, 293–5.
43. Carr ND, Mercey D, Slack WW. Non-condylomatous perianal disease in homosexual men. *Br J Surg* 1989; **76**:1064–6.
44. Van Calck M, Motte S, Rickaert F, Serruys E, Adler M, Wybran J. Cryptococcal anal ulceration in a patient with AIDS. *Am J Gastroenterol* 1988; **83**:1306–8.
45. Wexner SD. AIDS: what the colorectal surgeon needs to know. In Schrock T (ed), *Perspectives in Colon and Rectal Surgery* 1989; **2**(2): 19–54.

3

Pathophysiology of anoreceptive intercourse

Andrew JG Miles

Sexual orientation

There is considerable variation in the way in which the term 'homosexual' is interpreted. Some authors restrict the term to persons who have sexual contact with persons of the same sex, while others include sexual desires and fantasies towards persons of the same sex as well as overt sexual behaviour. In 1948, Kinsey and coworkers devised a numerical scale of sexual orientation based on both behaviour and fantasy (Table 3.1; [1]). This seven-point scale emphasizes the continuity of the spectrum of sexual orientation and recognizes that a person may shift his or her sexual orientation. Feldman and MacCulloch proposed a sub-classification of homosexuals into primary (those who have never experienced heterosexual arousal at any stage of their lives) and secondary (those who have experienced noticeable heterosexual arousal) [2]. They also maintained that with increasing age secondary homosexuals polarize, becoming either exclusively homosexual or exclusively heterosexual, with a decreasing proportion remaining bisexual.

A more useful definition of homosexuality was provided by Marmour and Green, who stated that 'homosexuality can be best described as a strong preferential attraction to members of the same sex' [3]. This definition does not include persons who indulge in anoreceptive intercourse whilst in unusual settings, such as prison or other single-sex institutions, as they are not generally regarded as homosexual by psychologists. However, they may present to the proctologist with pathology more usually associated with

Table 3.1   The Kinsey heterosexual/homosexual rating scale

0	Exclusively heterosexual
1	Predominantly heterosexual: only incidentally homosexual
2	Predominantly heterosexual: more than incidentally homosexual
3	Equally heterosexual and homosexual
4	Predominantly homosexual: more than incidentally heterosexual
5	Predominantly homosexual: only incidentally heterosexual
6	Exclusively homosexual

homosexuals. A working definition for the proctologist who is more concerned with problems arising from the physical act of anoreceptive intercourse than the psychology of homosexuality is that a male homosexual is a man who indulges in regular anoreceptive penile intercourse.

Numbers

The Kinsey survey was carried out more than 30 years ago, but to date it is the most extensive survey ever carried out. Interview data from 5300 white males in the report revealed that 4% were exclusively homosexual from puberty (7.4% at age 15), 10% were predominantly homosexual for at least three years between the ages of 16 and 55, and 37% had at least one homosexual experience leading to orgasm after the time of puberty. Although the results of this study may have been affected by a selection bias, as the samples were not random, in a study of sexual behaviour of teenagers in Britain during the early 1960s Schofield did not record any data regarding homosexual behaviour; and hence the Kinsey data remains the only large-scale study of male homosexuality.

Patterns of anoreceptive intercourse

Sexual gratification

Insertion of the penis into the anal canal is not physiological. It is a purely erotic maneuver that is practiced by a number of men and women. The anatomic basis of sexual gratification by anoreceptive intercourse (ARI) is the abundance of sensory endings in the anal canal, perineum, prostate, seminal vesicles and bladder which share afferent pathways with sensory endings from the external genitalia [4]. An erection of the penis may be produced by either tactile stimulation by the anus or voluntary contractions of the external anal sphincter. Similarly, stimulation of the genitals causes reflex contraction of the external anal sphincter; and contraction of the external anal sphincter occurs during orgasm, the anal contractions occurring simultaneously with the expulsive penile contractions of ejaculation [5].

Anal masturbation

Anal masturbation may be defined as anal self-manipulation in order to derive erotic sensations. This self-manipulation may be digital or may involve the insertion of objects. It may be performed at the same time as genital stimulation or may be performed on its own [6]. There are numerous reports of the variety of objects that are used for anal masturbation [7–9]. The objects are as varied as the maneuvers described for removing them after they have become lodged within the rectum [10].

Colonic irrigation may be used as a form of anal masturbation either consciously or subconsciously [11,12], and some individuals reach orgasm as a result of the peristaltic waves stimulated by enemata [13]. Anal masturbation has been proposed as the underlying cause for obsessive bowel consciousness and the persistent use of enemas and laxatives in some persons who have no demonstrable physical abnormality [14,15]. Enemas may also be used for the administration of recreational drugs or to wash or lubricate the rectum prior to anoreceptive intercourse.

Female anoreceptive intercourse

This chapter is primarily concerned with male homosexuals, but it should be borne in mind that ARI is also practiced by women as a method of contraception. In a survey of 100 000 married women published by *Redbook Magazine*, 43% of women had tried ARI at some time and 2% practiced it regularly [16]. It is likely that, before the advent of reliable and readily available contraception, ARI was practiced by women far more often. No studies have been published on the effect of anoreceptive intercourse on anorectal physiology in women.

Non-anoreceptive male homosexuals

Some homosexual men regard themselves as predominantly active partners in ARI and are not anally receptive themselves. This situation is much more frequent in the USA than in the UK, where most homosexual men are both active and passive. Thus when studying anorectal physiology in male homosexuals we have concentrated on males who have anoreceptive intercourse regularly.

Promiscuity

In the past, homosexuality has been associated with promiscuity. This association does not hold true for all male homosexuals but a proportion of the homosexual population have had large numbers of sexual partners. In a survey of men attending a medical genitourinary outpatient clinic, over 50% of homosexuals reported in excess of 100 partners in anoreceptive intercourse and 20% more than 1000 partners, whereas only 3% of heterosexuals reported more than 100 partners and none reported more than 1000 partners. The spread of the human immunodeficiency virus (HIV) has had a dramatic effect on sexual habits amongst male homosexuals and, in the future, it may not be reasonable to assume that male homosexuals will have had more sexual partners than male heterosexuals.

Anal trauma

It has been suggested that anal intercourse between consenting partners can be performed safely provided there is adequate lubrication, but that 'forceful anal penetration against a resistant sphincter will result in abrasive trauma, causing fissures, contusions, thrombosed hemorrhoids, lacerations with bleeding, pain and psychic trauma' [17]. The first statement is entirely reasonable as a great many persons of both sexes are known to have regular anoreceptive intercourse whilst few seek medical treatment for injuries thus sustained. The second statement may be true, although the authors provide no evidence to substantiate their opinions. While one can easily agree that contusion, fissure and laceration are quite possible outcomes of forced anal dilatation, the observation that thrombosed hemorrhoids might result is less easy to entertain. Indeed, one treatment for prolapsed hemorrhoids is manual dilatation of the anus [18].

The majority of injuries result from the insertion of large objects into the rectum [7–10]. The passage of such objects involves considerable dilatation of the sphincter muscles encircling the anal canal. (The increase in circumference of the anal canal, and hence in the length of the anal sphincters, being approximately three times the diameter of the object passed.) Whilst the external anal sphincter may be relaxed voluntarily the internal anal sphincter cannot. During defecation the internal anal sphincter relaxes by local reflex inhibition to allow the passage of stools [19]. This reflex relaxation will not be present during the anal dilatation of anoreceptive intercourse. Indeed, stimulation of the perianal skin during ARI is more likely to stimulate reflex *contraction* of the external anal sphincter [15,20]. The passage of large objects produces the same injuries reported to occur with forced anal penetration [9,10]. The worst injuries are usually the result of the insertion of a partner's hand or arm (or more rarely two hands) into the rectum (fist fornication—'fisting'—or brachioproctic intercourse) [21,22]. This is an extreme form of anal eroticism which is practiced by an unknown number of male homosexuals. The most dangerous complication is perforation of either the rectum or more commonly the sigmoid colon. This injury has resulted in at least one fatality from Fournier's gangrene as a result of delayed presentation of low rectal perforation [10]. A more frequent injury is mucosal laceration and hemorrhage. The hemorrhage appears to stop spontaneously in most cases, rarely requiring either transfusion or suturing. Surprisingly perhaps, complete disruption of the anal sphincters with subsequent incontinence is a rare injury [7,9,10].

Thus anoreceptive intercourse may involve the insertion of a variety of objects of various diameters, and the range of anal dilatation to which homosexuals subject each other is extremely varied. While the average dilatation associated with penile ARI may not be greatly different from that required for defecation, in the absence of the protective reflexes normally present during defecation the disruptive effect on the sphincters is likely to be greater. Insertion of large objects into the anal canal will result in a much greater anal dilatation and hence a greater risk of damaging the sphincters than that caused by insertion of a penis.

Effect of ARI on continence

Repetitive trauma of the anal sphincters results in a reduction in efficiency of the continence mechanism. A questionnaire distributed to 150 consecutive patients at the author's medical genitourinary clinic (78 homosexual and 72 heterosexual) revealed that over 25% of the homosexuals had accidental bowel actions (compared with less than 3% of age- and sex-matched heterosexuals). These episodes of incontinence were not associated with an alteration in bowel habit as on average there was no difference in frequency of defecation or stool consistency between homosexuals and heterosexuals. However, amongst homosexuals with AIDS there was a much greater incidence of incontinence: 50% of homosexuals with AIDS reported frequent accidental bowel actions. This excess of incontinence in patients with AIDS almost certainly results from a combination of proctitis and diarrhoea [23] putting a greater strain on the already compromised continence mechanism [24].

The symptoms of incontinence were not confined to homosexuals who practice the more extreme forms of anoreceptive intercourse. Most of the homosexuals in this study had never had anoreceptive brachioproctic intercourse, and those who had did not have more frequent episodes of incontinence. The responses to this questionnaire were remarkably similar to those obtained by interview of 40 homosexuals and 18 heterosexuals. These interviews were conducted within the confines of a secure and friendly environment likely to have increased the likelihood of accurate responses [25] and confirmed the excess of incontinence among homosexuals.

Objective measurements of anorectal physiology

Anal resting pressure
Homosexuals have lower maximum anal resting pressures (measured by water-filled mini-balloon techniques) than age- and sex-matched hetero-

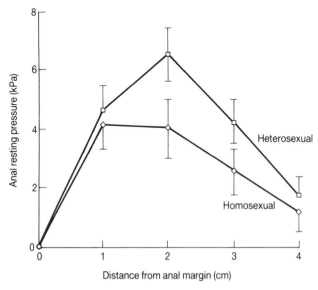

Figure 3.1 The resting pressure profile of the anal canal in homosexuals is significantly different ($p < 0.001$) from that of heterosexuals.

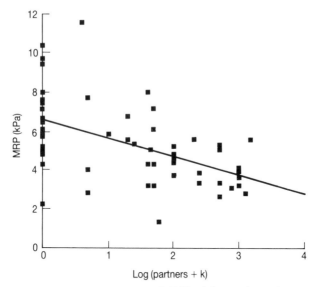

Figure 3.2 Maximum resting pressure (MRP) of the anal canal is inversely proportional ($r=-0.54$, $k=1$, $p<0.01$) to the logarithm of the number of partners that a homosexual has had during his lifetime.

sexuals [26]. The high-pressure zone is shorter, and the profile of anal sphincter resting pressure differs from that in heterosexuals (Fig. 3.1). The maximum anal resting pressure appears to be lower still in homosexuals who practice regular brachioproctic ARI, although we have only been able to study a small number of such homosexuals.

Damage to the internal anal sphincter, which is known to be responsible for 70% of the anal canal resting pressure [27], would explain this reduction in resting pressure observed in homosexuals. The concept of repeated local trauma damaging the sphincter is supported by the observation that the maximum resting pressure (MRP) is inversely proportional to the logarithm of the total number of partners with whom the homosexuals have been anoreceptive (Fig. 3.2). This correlation between maximum resting pressure and number of partners suggests that the damage to the internal sphincter is cumulative as homosexuals who report more partners are likely to have also had a greater number of anoreceptive episodes and hence more trauma to their sphincters. The lowest resting pressures are found in homosexuals who complain of incontinence for either flatus, liquid or solid stool (Fig. 3.3).

Voluntary anal squeeze pressure

Voluntary squeeze pressures are normal in continent homosexuals. Thus the observed reduction in anal resting pressure is not the result of reduced external anal sphincter function which normally contributes 15–25% of the anal resting pressure [28]. However, homosexuals who are incontinent have significantly lower maximum squeeze pressures (MSP) than homosexuals who have no symptoms of incontinence (Fig. 3.4).

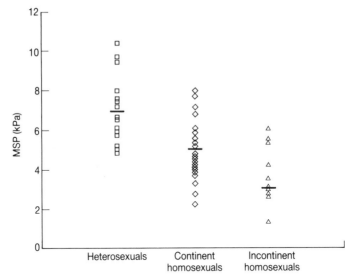

Figure 3.3 Maximum resting pressure (MRP) of the anal canal is significantly lower ($p < 0.01$) in continent homosexuals. Even lower pressures ($p < 0.01$) are found in homosexuals with incontinence of either flatus, liquid or solid stool.

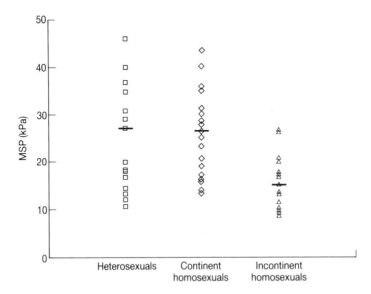

Figure 3.4 Maximum voluntary squeeze pressure (MSP) is significantly reduced ($p < 0.05$) in incontinent homosexuals but is normal in continent homosexuals.

Anal sensation

A reduction in anal sensation has been postulated as an important factor in the continence mechanism [29,30], and the threshold of anal mucosal electrosensitivity in homosexuals is higher than in heterosexuals [31]. However, this slight loss of anal sensitivity is much less than has been reported in other patient groups with incontinence and is not significantly greater in homosexuals with incontinence than in those who are fully continent. This reduction in anal sensitivity may be the result of repeated mucosal laceration and scarring, but it is unlikely that it is a major factor in the development of incontinence in homosexuals.

Rectal sensation

The threshold of rectal sensation to filling seems to be unaffected by anoreceptive intercourse as the volume of first constant sensation of rectal filling is not significantly different in homosexuals compared with hetero-sexuals (Fig. 3.5). Some homosexuals, especially those who practice brachioproctic intercourse ('fisting'), do have a much greater maximum tolerable rectal volume than normal (Fig. 3.5), which may either reflect a larger rectal capacity or possibly a higher pain threshold in homosexuals.

Pelvic floor

Perineal descent [32] is not excessive in homosexuals. The resting position of the perineum does not lie below the ischial tuberosities and does not balloon downwards on straining.

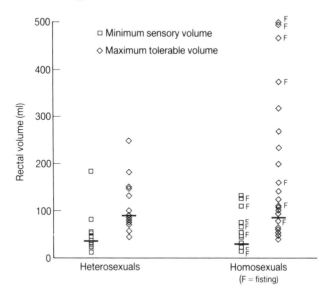

Figure 3.5   There is no significant difference in rectal sensation between homosexuals or heterosexuals, although some homosexuals have a much greater maximum tolerable volume, especially those who practice brachioproctic intercourse (fisting).

Peripheral neuropathy is well documented in AIDS [33] and may explain the increased incidence of incontinence in these patients. However, the pudendal nerve conduction times are normal, and the author's unit has been unable to find evidence of denervation by single-fibre EMG of the external anal sphincter in homosexuals who do not have AIDS.

Rectoanal inhibitory reflex

The rectoanal inhibitory reflex is dependant on intact local reflexes in the myenteric and submucosal nerve plexuses [34]. These nerve plexuses are not permanently disrupted by anoreceptive intercourse, the author's unit has been able to elicit the rectoanal inhibitory reflex in over 80% of homosexuals.

Reflex anal dilatation

Reflex anal dilatation has been described as a reliable indicator of anal penetration in chldren [35], although it has also been described in children with chronic constipation [36]. In the author's experience, spontaneous dilatation of the anal canal is not observed in adult homosexuals.

Animal studies on anal dilatation

The studies in male homosexuals suggest that the primary injury of anoreceptive intercourse is to the internal anal sphincter. *In vivo* experiments of the pharmacology of the internal anal sphincter have been performed in cats [37] and monkeys [38], and more recently the rat has been described as a suitable model for the investigation of internal anal sphincter physiology [39,40]. As in man, the internal anal sphincter of the rat is a continuation of the circular smooth muscle layer of the rectum. The external anal sphincter, which ends below the internal anal sphincter, is striated muscle, and ganglion cells have been observed both between the muscle layers (myenteric plexus) and in the submucosa [40]. Thus, as far as has been ascertained, the anatomy of the anal canal in the rat closely resembles that in man. Manometry of the anal canal has confirmed that slow waves, ultra-slow waves and the rectoanal inhibitory reflex are present [40].

The author's unit compared the effect of single and repeated anal dilatation to varying size in the rat. Having found that mean stool diameter for the rats prior to dilatation was 7 mm, we dilated groups of six rats for 60 seconds, either once to 7 mm, 9 mm or 11 mm or four times at 24 hours intervals to either 7 mm or 11 mm. We found that single dilatation to 11 mm, but not 7 mm or 9 mm, caused a significant reduction in anal pressure which returned to normal within 24 hours (Fig. 3.6). However, repeated dilatation to both 7 mm and 11 mm resulted in a significant reduction in anal pressure which did not recover within one month (Fig. 3.7). Thus in the animal model a single large dilatation produced a reduction in anal pressure, as has been observed in man [41], as did repeated dilatation to a diameter no greater

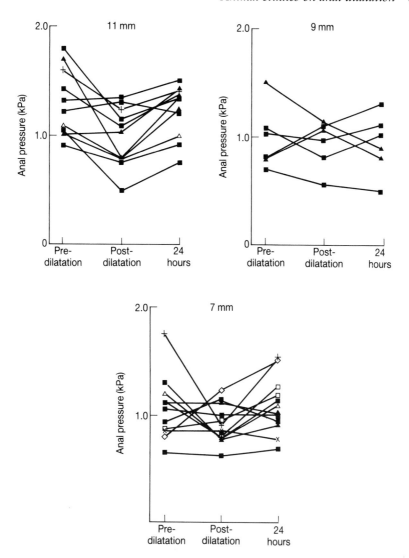

Figure 3.6 A single anal dilation to 11 mm but not 9 mm or 7 mm caused a significant reduction in anal pressure ($p < 0.01$) which had recovered to normal within 24 hours.

than that of normal stool, a situation analogous perhaps to anoreceptive intercourse.

Histology of the internal anal sphincter in these animals showed disruption of the smooth fibers and hemorrhage into the internal anal sphincter following the 11 mm dilatation. This resolved without scarring after only a single dilatation, but was associated with permanent abnormalities in the architecture of the internal anal sphincter in the animals which had repeated

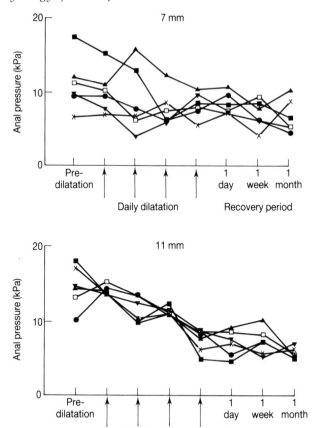

Figure 3.7   Four dilatations to either 7 mm or 11 mm at 24-hour intervals produced a significant reduction in resting pressure which had not recovered within one month.

dilatation to either 7 mm or 11 mm. It appears that permanent damage to the internal anal sphincter is related to the repetitive nature of the trauma, and this may be why homosexuals with the greatest number of partners have the lowest anal resting pressures.

Anorectal physiology and surgical management

In addition to sexually transmitted infections and conditions related to trauma, the anal canals of homosexuals are susceptive to the conditions encountered in heterosexual men, such as hemorrhoids, fissure and fistula [42], although the relative frequency of these conditions between the homosexual population and the heterosexual population is not known. The surgical management of these conditions must be modified to allow for the abnormalities of anal physiology present in homosexuals. Procedures

aimed at reducing internal sphincter activity, such as lateral internal sphincterotomy or manual dilatation, should not be performed in the absence of
objective evidence of internal anal sphincter spasm; and even then the risk
of impaired continence after the procedure is probably greater than for the
population in general. Similarly, caution should be exercised when treating
fistula-in-ano in order to avoid unacceptably high rates of postoperative
incontinence. We recommend sclerotherapy for hemorrhoids in preference
to surgical hemorrhoidectomy [43], as the reduction of anal sensation
following hemorrhoidectomy [44] may have a deleterious effect on the
continence of homosexuals.

With the exception of repair of acute traumatic rupture of the sphincters,
the author's unit has no experience of surgical correction of incontinence in
homosexuals. It would appear that while many homosexuals will admit to
incontinence when asked directly, relatively few are referred for treatment.
It is probably wise to advise incontinent homosexuals who seek treatment
against further damage to the internal anal sphincter by anoreceptive
intercourse, although this is unlikely to improve continence as homosexuals
who have abstained from ARI for some years do not have significantly
higher anal pressures than active homosexuals. Continence has been shown
to be related to stool consistency in other patients with incontinence [45]
and, as many of the homosexuals in our unit have AIDS with opportunistic
infection of the gut causing watery motions, constipating agents are the
mainstay of treatment of incontinence in these patients.

Conclusions

Anoreceptive intercourse is associated with reduced anal canal resting
pressure and an increased risk of minor fecal incontinence. These minor
defects of anal continence are similar to those that have been reported in
35% of patients following internal sphincterotomy [46] and manual dilatation of the anal canal [41]. Although therapeutic manual dilatation of the
anal canal involves much greater stretching than is produced by an erect
penis, which is of similar dimension to a large stool, passage of stool through
the anal canal is facilitated by reflex relaxation of the internal sphincter and
this protective mechanism may not be present during the forced dilatation of
ARI. Animal studies have confirmed that anal dilatation can cause hemorrhage into the internal anal sphincter and rupture of the smooth muscle
fibers, and a sustained reduction in internal anal sphincter function can
be produced by repeated dilatation of the anus to the same diameter as
fresh stool. Direct trauma to the internal anal sphincter during ARI is therefore the most likely cause of the reduced anal resting pressure abserved in
homosexuals.

The correlation between maximum resting pressure and estimated number of partners suggests that the damage to the internal sphincter is either a
cumulative effect or that the more promiscuous AR subjects practice more
traumatic forms of ARI. The small subgroup of 'fisters' that we have been
able to study did have significantly lower resting pressures when compared
with other, non-fisting homosexuals. However, the homosexuals who

practiced brachioproctic intercourse (fisting) also tended to have had large numbers of partners so that it is unclear which of these factors was responsible for their low anal resting pressures.

We have not observed the reflex anal dilatation in adult anoreceptive subjects which has been proposed as a sign of ARI in children [35], but the results of this study provide grounds for concern that anal interference in children could result in reduced internal anal sphincter function. The findings also suggest that repeated anal dilatation in other situations (for example, complete rectal prolapse or chronic constipation) may be damaging to the internal anal sphincter.

There are alternative explanations for the symptoms we have observed. Chronic proctitis or previous infections may be responsible for incontinence by reducing rectal compliance. Although the size of the rectal reservoir and not rectal compliance was assessed, it is unlikely that rectal compliance is reduced in homosexuals as assessment of rectal volume did not demonstrate reduced rectal capacity in homosxuals. Furthermore, if proctitis is the cause of the incontinence, homosexuals with incontinence would be expected to have more frequent defecation and a more liquid stool consistency. Another possibility is that a peripheral neuropathy affecting the pudendal nerves or cauda equina is responsible for the incontinence. Viral infections such as HIV or herpes simplex are known to affect the peripheral or central nervous systems. This might lead to fecal incontinence by denervation of the pelvic floor. However, we found no evidence of reduced anal or rectal sensation in the AR subjects and both anal voluntary squeeze pressure and perineal descent were normal.

The pathophysiology of the anus and rectum in male homosexuals is more consistent with internal anal sphincter damage than any other of the hypotheses. It is unlikely that anoreceptive subjects will abstain from ARI because of a small risk of future fecal incontinence. The importance of these findings is their relevance to surgery of the anus and rectum in homo- sexuals. Anorectal disease has become the most frequent reason for surgical referral of HIV-infected homosexuals [43,47] and an understanding of the pre-morbid anorectal physiology assists decision making when selecting the most appropriate treatment for these conditions.

References

1. Kinsey AC, Pomeroy WB, Martin CE. *Sexual Behaviour in the Human Male.* Philadelphia: WB Saunders, 1948.
2. Feldman MP, MacCulloch MJ. *Homosexual Behaviour: Therapy and Assessment.* Oxford: Pergamon, 1971.
3. Marmour J, Green R. Homosexual behavior. In: Money J and Musaph H (eds), *Handbook of Sexology.* New York: Elsevier/North Holland Biomedical Press, 1977: 1051–68.
4. Guyton AC. *Textbook of Medical Physiology.* Philadelphia: WB Saunders, 1981.
5. Masters WH, Johnson VE. *Human Sexual Response.* Boston: Little Brown, 1966.
6. Katchadourian HA, Lunde DT. *Fundamentals of Human Sexuality.* New York: Holt, Rinehart & Winston, 1972.

7. Crass RA, Tranbaugh RF, Kudsk KA. Colorectal foreign bodies and perforation. *Am J Surg* 1981; **142**:85–8.
8. Eftaiha M, Hambrick E, Abcarain H. Principles of management of colo-rectal foreign bodies. *Arch Surg* 1977; **112**:691–5.
9. Sohn N, Weinstein MA, Gonchar J. Social injuries of the rectum. *AM J Surg* 1977; **134**:611–12.
10. Barone JE, Yee JK, Nealon TF. Management of foreign bodies and trauma of the rectum. *Surg Gynaecol Obstet* 1983; **156**:543–7.
11. Denko JD. Klismaphilia: enema as a sexual preference. *Am J Psychotherapy* 1973; **27**:232.
12. Rowan RL, Gillette PJ. *The Gay Health Guide*. Boston: Little Brown, 1978.
13. Greenberg-Englander S, Levine S. Significance of frequent enemas. *Med Aspects Hum Sexual* 1981; **15**:116.
14. Caprio F. *Variations in Sexual Behaviour*. New York: Grove Press, 1955.
15. Agnew J. Some anatomical and physiological aspects of anal sexual practices. *J Homosex* 1986; **12**:75–96.
16. Tavris C, Sadd S. *The Redbook Report on Female Sexuality*. New York: Delacorte Press, 1975.
17. Bush RA, Owen RA. Trauma and other non-infectious problems in homosexual men. *Med Clin N Am* 1986; **70** (3):549–66.
18. Lord PH. *Proc R Soc Med* 1968; **61**:935.
19. Read NW, Timms JM. Defaecation and the pathophysiology of constipation. *Clin Gatroenterol* 1986; **15** (4): 937–65.
20. Melzac J, Porter NH. Studies of the reflex activity of the external anal sphincter ani in spinal man. *Paraplegia* 1964; **1**:277–96.
21. Lowry TP, Williams GR. Brachioproctic eroticism. *Br J Sex Med* 1981; **8**:32–3.
22. Shook LL, Whittle R, Rose EF. Rectal fist insertion—an unusual form of sexual behaviour. *Am J For Med Pathol* 1985; **6** (4): 319–24.
23. Weller IVD. ABC of AIDS: gastro-intestinal and hepatic manifestations. *Br Med J* 1987; **294**:174–6.
24. Read NW, Harford WV, Schumulen AC, Read MG, Ana CS, Fordtran JS. A clinical study of patients with fecal incontinence and diarrhea. *Gastroenterology* 1979; **76**:747–56.
25. Bauman KA, Hale FA. Bringing the homosexual patient out: teaching the doctor's role. *Med-Educ* 1985; **19** (6): 459–62.
26. Miles AJG, Allen-Mersh TG, Wastell C. The damaging and cumulative effect of ano-receptive intercourse on internal anal sphincter function. *Br J Surg* 1990 (abstract) (in press).
27. Lester B, Penninckx FC, Kerremans R. The composition of anal basal pressure. *Int J Colorect Dis* 1989; **4**:118–28.
28. Frenckner B, Von Euler C. Influence of pudendal block on the function of the anal sphincters. *Gut* 1975; **16**:482–9.
29. Rogers J, Henry MM, Misiewicz JJ. Combined sensory and motor deficit in primary neuropathic faecal incontinence. *Gut* 1988; **29**:5–9.
30. Miller R, Bartolo DCC, Cervero F, Mortensen NJMcC. Anorectal temperature sensation: a comparison of normal and incontinent patients. *Br J Surg* 1987; **74**:511–15.
31. Roe AM, Bartolo DCC, Mortensen NJMcC. New method for assessment of anal sensation in various anorectal disorders. *Br J Surg* 1986; **73**:310–12.
32. Henry MM, Parks AG, Swash M. The pelvic floor musculature in the descending perineum syndrome. *Br J Surg* 1982; **69**:470–72.
33. Guiloff RJ, Fuller GN, Roberts A, Hargreaves M, Gazzard B, Scaravti JN, Hare W. The nature incidence and prognosis of neurological involvement in the

acquired immunodeficiency syndrome in central London. *Post Grad Med J* 1988; **64**:919–25.

34. Lawson JON, Nixon HH. Anal canal pressure in the diagnosis of Hirschprung's disease. *J Paediat Surg* 1967; **2**:544–8.
35. Hobbs CJ, Wynne JM. Buggery in childhood—a common syndrome of child abuse. *Lancet* 1986; **ii**:792–6.
36. Claydon STH. RAD in constipation. Personal communication.
37. Garrett JR, Howard ER, Jones W. The internal anal sphincter in the cat: a study of nervous mechanisms affecting tone and reflex activity. *J Physiol Lond* 1974; **286**:153–66.
38. Rayner V. Characteristics of the internal anal sphincter and rectum in the vervet monkey. *J Physiol Lond* 1979; **286**:383–99.
39. Nissan S, Vinograd I, Hadary AK, Merguerian P, Zamir O, Lernau OZ, Hanani M. Physiological and pharmacological studies of the internal anal sphincter in the rat. *J Paediat Surg* 1984; **19**:12–14.
40. Vinogrand Il, Hanini M, Handary A, Merguerian P, Nissan S. Animal Model for the study of internal anal sphincter activity. *Eur Surg Res* 1985; **17**:259–63.
41. Hancock BD. Measurement of anal pressure and motility. *Gut* 1976; **17**:645–51.
42. Kazal HL, Sohn N, Carrasco JI, Robilotti JG, Delaney WE. The gay bowel syndrome: clinico-pathologic correlation in 260 cases. *Ann Clin Lab Sci* 1976; **6**:184–92.
43. Miles AJG, Mellor CH, Gazzard BG, Allen-Mersh TG, Wastell C. Surgical management of anorectal disease in HIV-positive homosexuals. *Br J Surg* 1990; **77**:869–71.
44. Read MG, Read NW, Haynes WG, Donnelly TC, Johnson AG. A prospective study of the effects of haemorrhoidectomy on sphincter function and anal continence. *Br J Surg* 1982; **69**:396–8.
45. Read NW, Timms JM. Defaecation and the pathophysiology of constipation. *Clin Gastroenterol* 1986; **15** (4):937–65.
46. Khubchandani IT, Reed JF. Sequelae of sphincterotomy for chronic fissure-in-ano. *Br J Surg* 1989; **76**:431–4.
47. Wexner SD, Smithy WB, Milson JW, Daily TH. The surgical management of anorectal diseases in AIDS and preAIDS patients. *Dis Colon Rectum* 1986; **29**:719–23.

EXAMINATION

4

Precautions when managing the HIV-infected patient
Timothy I Davidson and Timothy G Allen-Mersh

There can be no doubt that additional precautionary measures should be taken when examining and treating HIV-positive patients. At present, routine preoperative screening of patients for HIV has not been accepted as general surgical practice [1,2]. In the majority of patients presenting to the clinician, therefore, the HIV status will be unknown. There is no universal agreement as to which patients should be treated as 'at risk'. Broadly speaking, there are two points of view: on the one hand that universal precautions should be adopted in *all* patients (i.e. as though they were HIV positive), and on the other hand that attempts should be made to identify those patients most likely to be at risk.

Identifying patients at risk

In the USA clinicians from areas with a high prevalence of HIV disease—such as New York and San Francisco—maintain that all patients should be treated as HIV-positive until proven otherwise [3]. The argument for assuming every patient to be a potential HIV carrier, and therefore for exercising *universal precautions*, means that such precautions are taken regardless of the patient's HIV status or of known risk factors. The window of HIV seronegativity can vary from three weeks to more than three years [4], and thus surgeons who rely on the HIV test to identify 'at risk' patients may expose themselves to unnecessary risk. Because neither clinical history, physical examination nor laboratory data can identify all HIV-infected patients, the Centers for Disease Control (CDC) has advocated exercising universal precautions for all patients whether or not they have known risk factors, are HIV-positive or have AIDS [5,6]. This has now been adopted as standard practice in centers with a high prevalence of HIV, but the practice of surgeons treating anorectal disease in low-prevalence areas of the USA is less well documented.

In the UK, current practice is to attempt to identify patients at risk of HIV infection prior to undertaking any procedure [2,3]. Such 'at risk' groups include homosexuals, bisexuals, intravenous drug misusers, hemophiliacs, partners of people known to be HIV-positive and patients from high-prevalence areas such as sub-Saharan Africa. It is argued that in the UK the number of HIV infected persons outside one of the recognized risk groups is very small. The same precautions are taken with patients belonging to an 'at risk' group as those when treating patients known to be HIV-positive. In a patient considered to be at risk it must be borne in mind that a negative HIV antibody test does *not* exclude the possibilities that the patient has been infected with HIV after the test was performed, or may have been at CDC stage 1 infection (and hence be HIV antigen-positive but not have developed antibodies) at the time of testing.

The question of preoperative testing for HIV raises ethical and practical issues and its value in terms of reducing the risk to the surgeon has been questioned [1,2]. In the UK, the Royal College of Surgeons of Edinburgh has advocated preoperative testing for patients suspected of being infected with HIV, with the patient's consent in elective procedures but without it in emergencies [7]. The American Medical Association has likewise recommended patient screening in high-prevalence settings [8]. Central to the issue of preoperative testing are whether the risk to the clinician is reduced by the prior knowledge of the HIV status of the patient and whether the policy of adopting universal precautions is a practical and financially viable alternative. There may be disadvantages to the patient in preoperative HIV testing, and the rate of false-positive results, although small, must be borne in mind. Maintaining confidentiality is a further problem and HIV testing before an operation or examination may not be the best environment for counseling and dealing with the many complex problems that this raises.

As in the USA, most information on the awareness of HIV and its impact on surgical practices in the UK has come from centers in high-prevalence areas. Elsewhere in the UK, surgeons seem to have a low perception of exposure risk to HIV and currently take few additional precautions [9]. It would appear that prevailing attitudes are similar in Australia [10]. While present epidemiological evidence indicates HIV prevalence outside the defined risk groups to be very low in the UK, the two-tier practice of taking special precautions only for those identified as being 'at risk' is likely to continue. Clearly such a policy will no longer be acceptable once HIV is recognized to be a significant problem in the non-drug-user heterosexual population.

The magnitude of risk

Available data indicate that the risk to the clinician of becoming infected with HIV as a result of adverse exposure (needlestick or sharps injury, or mucous membrane exposure) is small [1,2,11]. Mucous membrane exposure has been very rarely implicated and occupational exposure from HIV-infected patients is from a sharps injury in about 90% of cases [11]. Injuries involving hollow needles or with actual inoculation of patient blood constitute the highest risk.

How great is the risk of seroconversion after a sharps injury? Combined surveillance studies from several centers [12] reported 16 seroconversions among more than 3200 people injured while working with HIV-infected material. Those most at risk seem to be nurses and there is circumstantial evidence in only four surgeons of seroconversion following occupational exposure [5].

The degree of risk to the surgeon depends on the caseload of HIV-positive patients. In high-prevalence (25–30%) areas the risk of seroconversion is estimated to be one infection every eight years [13]. In low-prevalence (< 3%) areas the estimated risk of seroconversion (based on 500 operations per year) is calculated at 1 in 800 for an occupational lifespan of 30 years [14]. A widely accepted estimate of risk for seroconversion following a single adverse exposure to HIV with a sharps injury is 4.2 per 1000, or roughly 0.5% [11].

To date only five cases of seroconversion have been reported following exposure of skin or mucous membranes to blood [15]. In Elista, Russia, 27 children were thought to have been infected with HIV as a result of poor infection control within the hospital [16]. The risk of transmission of HIV between patients and health workers in the absence of a recognized sharps injury is harder to quantify. It has, however, been postulated that the Langerhans cells in intact skin and mucous membrane are the primary target cells of sexually-transmitted HIV infection [17].

What body fluids constitute the greatest risk? In the UK the Department of Health [18] has recommended the use of universal precautions when dealing with blood and certain other body fluids (peritoneal, pleural, pericardial, amniotic fluid, semen, vaginal secretions or any body fluid containing visible blood). Such precautions have been deemed unnecessary when dealing with feces, sweat or urine. A routine and atraumatic anorectal examination therefore involves less potential risk exposure than an operative anorectal procedure. There is no evidence for fecal–oral spread of HIV and it appears unlikely that HIV could penetrate intact skin.

In considering occupational adverse exposure, risks from agents other than HIV must be considered. As with HIV, there is no evidence of transmission of hepatitis B virus (HBV) by the fecal–oral route or droplet inhalation, but the risk of HBV transmission following a sharps injury is high (up to 20%) following inoculation accidents involving HBsAg-positive blood [19]. Hepatitis A is spread by the fecal–oral route but carries substantially less risk in terms of morbidity and mortality.

Precautions in the clinic and operating room

A dedicated operating room or clinic examination area for 'at risk' cases, though often expedient, is not considered a necessary precaution, but the use of areas that are cramped or difficult to clean should be avoided. Operating theaters should contain the minimum amount of equipment required for each case. The operating table or examination couch should be covered with a plastic sheet.

For their own protection, operating room staff must know that the patient with known or suspected HIV is an 'at risk' or 'inoculation risk' patient, and the written operating list must be annotated accordingly. HIV-infected patients need not be scheduled to undergo surgery at the end of operating lists [2].

The number of attendant personnel should be kept to the minimum required for safe operating or to conduct the examination. Staff should be discouraged from leaving and entering the clinic or theater during a case. Procedures involving HIV-infected patients should be performed by fully trained medical and nursing staff. Because of their relative inexperience, medical students are vulnerable to sharps injuries [20] and the use of medical students and student nurses to help with HIV cases should be avoided.

Medical staff with cuts or abrasions should cover the areas with a waterproof plaster before entering the operating area. Staff with abrasions on their hands should be excluded from theater. All hospital staff should be immunized against hepatitis B.

Blood soak-through means that conventional linen gowns do not provide theater staff with an adequate barrier to the patient's blood [21] (see Chapter 5). Disposable theater gowns with plasticized, fluid-resistant reinforcement of sleeves and anterior body areas are ideal. Waterproof fabrics with the ability to 'breathe' are available and may prove more comfortable during lengthy operations. Disposable plastic aprons should be worn under gowns.

Boots offer better protection than clogs against blood spillage. Knee-high rubber boots have been introduced in some centers. Fenestrated footwear should not be worn because of the risk from a falling sharp instrument. Disposable overshoes are worn over the boots or clogs.

The importance of protecting against eye contamination from blood splashes has been emphasized [22] and staff working in close proximity to the operating area must wear a visor, or safety glasses or goggles (Fig. 4.1) which afford better protection than ordinary spectacles. Eye protection must be either disposable or must be cleaned and disinfected after use.

The use of surgical gloves as a mechanical barrier to HIV is universally accepted [23] and the wearing of double gloves to further reduce the incidence of hand contamination by body fluids has been adopted in many centers [2]. The use of double-gloving will not reduce the incidence of needlestick injuries (and some have argued may even increase this because of impairment of dexterity) but reduces the incidence of inadvertent glove perforation [24–26]. As soon as a perforation of one or both layers of gloves is recognized, they should be discarded and the surgeon should re-glove. The merits of double gloving are discussed in greater detail in Chapter 5.

Precautions with rigid endoscopes

The use of disposable plastic anoscopes and rectoscopes (below, Fig. 4.2) will avoid the need for instrument cleaning and the additional exposure to the staff involved in such cleaning. Reusable metal instruments must be thoroughly cleaned of all debris with soap and water prior to sterilization by autoclaving or gas sterilization. Handling of such instruments during clean-

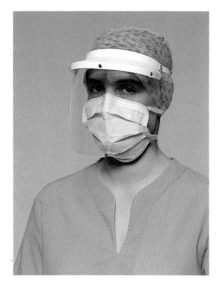

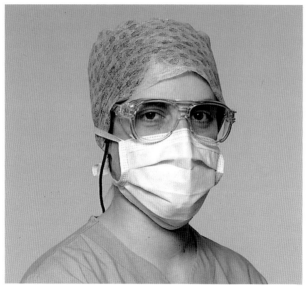

Figure 4.1 Disposable visor (above) or goggles (below) should be worn by staff working in close proximity to an HIV-positive patient undergoing operation.

ing must not be left to untrained staff and surgical or household gloves must be worn. After cleaning, the metal endoscopes must be sealed in prominently marked containers and returned to the central sterile supply department for sterilization.

Care must be taken when performing injections or other procedures through rigid endoscopes. As with sharp instruments in all hospital practice, needles should not be resheathed after use. A significant number of

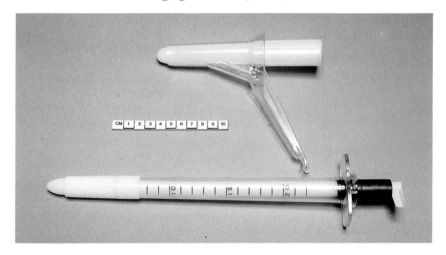

Figure 4.2   Disposable plastic anoscope (above) and rectoscope (below) for use in anorectal examination of HIV-positive patients.

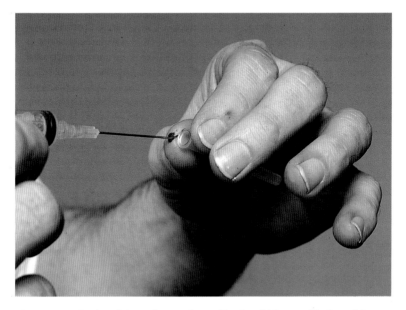

Figure 4.3   Resheathing of a used needle should be avoided as this may result in inadvertent stabbing of the thumb or index finger.

sharps injuries occur while resheathing needles (Fig. 4.3) and this should be avoided. It is the personal responsibility of the individual using a sharp instrument to dispose of it safely in a rigid combustible sharp container and disposal should not be left for others to do. In anorectal patients special care must be taken with the handling of sclerotherapy needles, and the use of spiked forceps for rectal biopsy is unnecessary and hazardous.

Precautions with fiber-optic endoscopes

Because they are not disposable and not autoclavable, fiber-optic endoscopes require special precautions during and after their use in examining the patient with HIV.

The British Society of Gastroenterology has recommended that all patients be considered at risk and that adequate antibacterial and antiviral disinfection is needed before and after each GI endoscopy [27]. A two-tier system of cleaning and disinfection, or the use of a dedicated instrument for HIV-positive patients, is not recommended. Thorough manual physical cleaning of the endoscope internally and externally with detergent before disinfection is the most important part of the cleaning procedure. A disinfectant will be ineffective if micro-organisms are shielded from contact by organic material.

Aldehyde preparations (2% activated alkaline gluteraldehyde, Cidex, and related products) are the recommended first-line antibacterial and antiviral disinfectant. A 4-minute soak is sufficient for inactivation of vegetative bacteria and viruses including HBV and HIV. Other aldehyde preparations such as Gigasept 10% are considered less irritant and allergenic and are probably equally effective as an antiviral disinfectant. Because of the high sensitivity to aldehyde disinfectants, suitable exhaust extraction facilities such as hoods or cabinets or closed-circuit washing machines should be provided in work areas. In addition to gloves, suitable eye protection should be provided where splashing might occur.

Quaternary ammonium detergents (8% Dettox for 2 minutes for bacterial disinfection) followed by exposure of the endoscope shaft and channels to ethyl alcohol (70% for 4 minutes for viral inactivation) is an acceptable second-line disinfection routine where staff sensitization prevents the use of an aldehyde disinfectant. At San Francisco General Hospital, flexible endoscopes are cleaned and sterilized with peroxyacetic acid as a sterilizing fluid (total time for sterilization 19 minutes) [3].

Cleaning and disinfection of flexible endoscopes is a specialized procedure which should be carried out only by staff who have been properly trained. The disinfection procedure should be performed prior to use, between each patient examined, and at the end of the list. Longer periods of disinfection (> 20 minutes) are recommended at the end of the list to reduce the risk of bacterial growth during storage. Endoscope channels (especially the air channel) must be washed free of any refluxed mucus or proteinaceous material and brushes and other cleaning equipment must themselves be disinfected or sterilized before each use. It is recommended that the use of non-immersible endoscopes be discontinued because of difficulties in ensuring adequate cleaning.

Although HIV transmission via the fecal–oral route has not been demonstrated, possible contamination of the clinician with fecal fluid expelled during both rigid and fiber-optic endoscopy can occur. The availability of a camera attachment and video monitor will allow the endoscopist's face to be kept away from the field with less chance of exposure to fecal fluid with insufflation of the lumen during the examination.

Precautions during surgical procedures

Sharps injuries constitute the most important risk of exposure to HIV. Meticulous attention must be given at all times to the handling and disposal of sharp instruments, and operative technique modified. Sharp instruments, either scalpel or mounted needle, should not be passed directly between scrub nurse, assistant or operator. Sharp instruments should be placed into and retrieved from a receiver dish or basin (Fig. 4.4). Only one scalpel at a time is placed in the basin.

When handling tissues, a 'no-touch' technique should be used wherever possible. Hand-held needles should not be used. When placing sutures the tissues should be supported with forceps and not fingers. The commonest site for perforation of surgical gloves and needlestick injury is the index finger of the non-dominant hand (see Chapter 5). The use of a thimble over this finger to minimize the risk has been advocated but is not widely practiced.

Electrocautery dissection reduces the use of sharp instruments and has the added advantage of minimizing capillary bleeding. The use of skin strips (suture strips) and tissue adhesive glue and skin staples will reduce the need for skin suturing. When tying sutures by hand the needle should first be removed.

Although gowns, gloves and protective eye-wear will reduce the contamination of the surgeon's skin and mucous membranes by the patient's blood or body fluids, the standard surgical mask will not prevent inhalation of electrocautery smoke or aerosols if generated during the procedure. The possible risk of HIV transmission via aerosols has been of particular concern in orthopedic procedures because of the use of power tools, and high-pressure irrigation systems [28]. The low occupational risk of dentists who are heavily exposed to aerosols is, however, reassuring [29].

The demonstrated transmission of intact viral DNA from human papilloma virus (HPV) by a laser-generated plume of smoke following vaporization of genital wart tissue [30,31] has raised concern. In anorectal surgery this may have particular relevance to potential smoke inhalation during the use of electrocautery for hemostasis, or the treatment of perianal warts (see Chapter 10) by electrocautery or carbon-dioxide laser with a theoretical risk of transmission of both HIV and HPV. An efficient smoke evacuator should be used to scavenge electrocautery or laser smoke into a suitable filtration system.

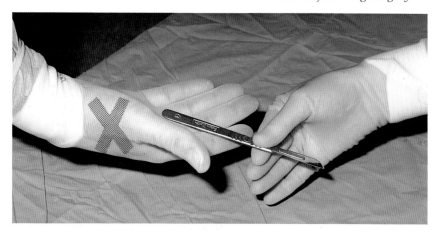

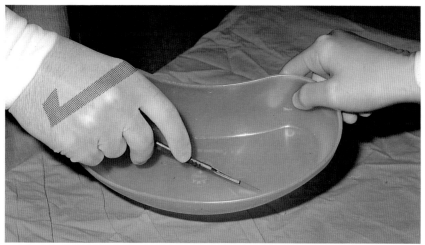

Figure 4.4 The scrub nurse and surgeon should not pass sharp instruments from hand to hand (above). One instrument only should be placed in a receiver which is then held so that the operating surgeon can remove the instrument from the receiver and replace it when it is no longer required (below).

Precautions following surgery

Removal of or changing the outer pair of gloves at the end of the procedure when applying dressings to the wound will avoid blood contamination on the outer surface of the dressing. Nursing and auxiliary staff in theater, in the recovery area and on the ward will need to take appropriate care to avoid contamination from the dressing or wound area.

At the end of the procedure the patient drapes, surgeons' gowns, over-shoes, gloves and safety glasses, masks or visors are collected for sub-sequent disposal in sealed plastic bags as the staff leave the theater area. Gloves and protective clothing must be worn by the staff involved in cleaning and disposal procedures. Disposable liners for suction bottles are the preferred method of handling operative and endoscopic suction waste, the filled and sealed bags being sent for incineration. Following a surgical procedure instruments are cleaned in soap and water and then placed in a clearly marked autoclavable bag. The instruments are then autoclaved in the central sterile supply department, repacked and re-autoclaved.

Following the operative procedure, blood and body fluid spillages on the operating table or floor are cleaned with sodium hypochlorite (bleach) or sodium dichloroisocyanurate (Presept) in concentrations of 10000 ppm available chlorine. The whole area should then be cleaned with a general-purpose detergent and boots and clogs should be cleaned with hypochlorite or Presept at the end of each case if they are contaminated.

When taking biopsy specimens for histologic or microbiologic examination, the risk to laboratory staff must be borne in mind. Immersion of tissue in formaldehyde or formol saline fixative causes rapid inactivation of HIV. Unfixed tissues should be handled with the same precautions as blood [18] and tissue specimens for histologic examination should be sent in fixative whenever possible. The pathology department should be informed when unfixed tissue is being sent. Specimen jars and forms should be clearly labelled to indicate inoculation risk, and sealed in plastic bags.

Precautions following adverse exposure to HIV

Following adverse exposure to blood or body fluids from a patient with HIV, the advised code of practice should be followed [32]. In the first instance the type of exposure and the consequent degree of risk should be assessed. The least risk is implicated by mucous membrane or skin exposure where no breach or ulceration in the skin exists. A superficial sharps injury to the skin (e.g. with a scalpel blade) is considered intermediate risk. The greatest risk is carried by a deep or intramuscular sharps injury, a hollow needlestick injury, or a massive exposure involving large-volume injection (> 1 ml) of a patient's blood.

Immediately following a sharps injury, the clinician should encourage bleeding and wash the area under running water. Sharps injuries should be reported immediately, an incident report filed, and the injured member of staff seen for advice and treatment by the occupational health department or other relevant body. With simple mucous membrane exposure (for instance a blood splash to the eyes) no specific treatment is advised apart from standard irrigation with eyewash.

Following a high-risk sharps injury immediate prophylactic zidovudine (AZT) is now advised [33,34]. Zidovudine 1 g orally should be given without delay, followed by 200 mg 4–6 hourly orally for 2–4 weeks [35,36]. Zidovudine carries dose-related side-effects, its long-term toxicity is not known, and seroconversion has occurred despite zidovudine prophylaxis [37]. The benefits of zidovudine prophylaxis do not clearly outweigh its risks when given after exposure to blood of unknown serological status or if there is a delay in starting therapy [36].

Without delaying the commencement of zidovudine prophylaxis, the exposed clinician may after counseling wish to ascertain his own serological status and confirm or exclude subsequent seroconversion. The injured member of staff should have blood taken with informed consent for storage and possible future testing. Blood from the source patient should be tested with informed consent for HIV and HBV. If the source patient is found to be HIV-negative, prophylactic zidovudine may be discontinued. If the patient is HIV-positive the injured member of staff is advised to have HIV testing 3 months later. An initial HIV-negative test followed by documented sero-conversion within the 3-month period following adverse exposure is taken to be indicative of occupationally acquired HIV disease. The full personal and professional implications of undergoing the HIV test at both stages needs to be discussed with trained counsellors.

If the source patient is found to be HBV-positive and the immune status of the injured staff is inadequate, a course of hepatitis B immunoglobulin should be instituted without delay. In hepatitis B, 10^{13} infectious particles may be present in each milliliter, compared with only 10^4/ml for HIV [38]; hence the far greater infectivity of HBV compared with HIV must be borne in mind.

Protection of the HIV-infected patient

Although precautions when examining and treating the patient with HIV are in the main designed to protect the clinician and ancillary healthcare workers, it must be remembered that the patient with HIV disease may have special psychological, physical and immunological problems which require special attention and precautions. Patients with AIDS may have severe wasting of body mass and may experience discomfort on the examination couch or operating table during lengthy procedures without general anesthesia. Special care must be taken over pressure areas.

There have been no long-term studies on the immunological response of HIV-infected patients to surgery. Major surgery and general anesthesia in HIV-negative patients is associated with a transient (3–6 day) depression of cell-mediated immunity [39] which does not affect outcome. However, there has been concern that surgical intervention may accelerate the progression of HIV disease [40]. This question remains unresolved, but provides a further reason to avoid unnecessary surgery or anesthesia in the patient with HIV infection.

Impairment of wound healing in the anorectal and other areas has been reported in HIV patients and may influence or alter the surgeon's management. Similarly, the high prevalence of diarrhea and associated minor fecal incontinence in patients with HIV disease should discourage the clinician from performing anal stretch in favor of alternative management. The question of anal sphincter damage is discussed in further detail in Chapter 3.

The immunocompromised state and susceptibility to infection in the HIV patient must be considered when performing simple anorectal examination and endoscopy [8]. Fiber-optic endoscopes should be immersed for a full hour in gluteraldehyde 2% prior to use to ensure, firstly, that opportunistic organisms such as atypical mycobacteria or cryptosporidia are not transmitted from one immunocompromised patient to another, and secondly, that *M. tuberculosis* is not transmitted from asymptomatic patient with HIV infection to an immunocompetent patient.

Because of their immune deficiency, patients with HIV disease undergoing anorectal surgery should be given systemic antibiotic prophylaxis to prevent bacteremic complications. The antibacterial spectrum should include anaerobic and Gram-negative organisms. One suitable prophylactic regimen is metronidazole 500 mg IV and cefuroxime 750 mg IV given with induction of anesthesia prior to the commencement of the anorectal procedure.

Finally, care must be taken with regard to the psychological needs of these patients who have a fatal disease. Despite the extensive range of precautions that need to be taken at every stage when examining and treating the patient with known or suspected HIV infection, the relationship between surgeon and patient must remain unaltered. The obligation of the clinician to manage his patient to the best of his or her ability must continue, and the need for additional precautions outlined in this chapter must not break the relationship of trust, compassion and confidentiality between doctor and patient.

References

1. Hagen MD, Klemens B, Meyer MD, Pauker SG. Routine preoperative screening for HIV: does the risk to the surgeon outweigh the risk to the patient? *JAMA* 1988; **259**:1357–9.
2. Gazzard BG, Wastell C. HIV and surgeons. *Br Med J* 1990; **301**:1003–4.
3. Gottesman LG, Miles AJ, Milsom JW *et al.* The management of anorectal disease in HIV-positive patients (clinical conference). *Int J Colorect Dis* 1990; **5**:61–72.
4. Lee MH, Waxman H, Gillooley JF. Primary malignant lymphoma of the anorectum in homosexual men. *Dis Colon Rectum* 1986; **29**:413–16.
5. Centers for Disease Control. Guidelines for prevention of transmission of human immunodeficiency virus and hepatitis B virus to health care and public safety workers. *MMWR* 1989; **38** (suppl S6).
6. Centers for Disease Control. Recommendations for prevention of HIV transmission in health care settings. *MMWR* 1987; **36** (suppl S2).
7. Royal College of Surgeons of Edinburgh. Statement to fellows on HIV infection and AIDS. Edinburgh, 1989.
8. Board of Trustees: Prevention and control of acquired immunodeficiency syndrome: an interim report. *JAMA* 1987; **258**:2097–103.
9. Stotter AT, Guillou PJ, Vipond MN. The response of general surgeons to HIV in England and Wales. *Ann Roy Coll Surg* 1990; **72**:251–6.
10. Jones ME. A thing about AIDS. *Anaesth Intens Care* 1989; **17**:253–63.
11. Marcus R. Centres for Disease Control Cooperative Needlestick Surveillance Group, Surveillance of health care workers exposed to blood from patients infected with the human immunodeficiency virus. *N Eng J Med* 1988; **319**:1118–23.
12. Barnes DM. Health workers and AIDS: questions persist. *Science* 1988; **241**:161–2.
13. Gerberding JL, Littell C, Tarkington A, Brown A, Schecter WP. Risk of exposure of surgical personnel to patients' blood during surgery at San Francisco General Hospital. *N Engl J Med* 1990; **322**:1788–93.
14. Leentvaar-Kuijpers A, Keeman JN, Dekker E *et al.* HIV: occupational risk of

surgical specialists and operation room personnel in the St Lucas Hospital in Amsterdam. *Ned Tijdschr Geneeskd* 1989; **133**:2388–91.

15. CDC Update: Human immunodeficiency virus infections in health-care workers exposed to blood of infected patients. *MMWR* 1987; **36**:285–9.

16. Belitsky N. Children infect mothers in AIDS outbreak at a Soviet hospital. *Nature* 1988; **337**:493.

17. Braathen LR *et al.* Langerhans cells as primary target cells for HIV infection. *Lancet* 1987; **2**:1094.

18. United Kingdom Departments of Health. Guidance for clinical health care workers. Recommendations of the expert advisory group on AIDS. HMSO, London, 1990.

19. Werner BG, Grady GF. Accidental hepatitis B surface-antigen-positive inoculations. *Ann Int Med* 1982; **97**:367–9.

20. Gompertz S. Needlestick injuries in medical students. *J Soc Occup Med* 1990; **40**: 19–20.

21. Closs JS, Tierney AJ. Theatre gowns: a survey of the extent of user protection. *J Hosp Infect* 1990; **15**: 375–8.

22. Duthie GS, Johnson SR, Packer GJ, Mackie IG. Eye protection, HIV, and orthopaedic surgery. *Lancet* 1988; **1**:481–82.

23. Dalgleish AG, Malkovsky M. Surgical gloves as a mechanical barrier against human immunodeficiency viruses. *Br J Surg* 1988; **75**:171–2.

24. Brough SF, Hunt TM, Barrie WW. Surgical glove perforations. *Br J Surg* 1988; **75**:317.

25. Matta H, Thompson AM, Rainey JB. Does wearing two pairs of gloves protect operating theatre staff from skin contamination: *Br Med J* 1988; **297**:597–8.

26. McLeod GG. Needlestick injuries at operations for trauma: are surgical gloves an effective barrier? *J Bone Joint Surg* 1989; **71**:489–91.

27. Working Party of the British Society of Gastroenterology. Cleaning and disinfection of equipment for gastrointestinal flexible endoscopy: interim recommendations. *Gut* 1988; **29**:1134–51.

28. American Academy of Orthopaedic Surgeons Task Force. Recommendations for the prevention of human immunodeficiency virus (HIV) transmission in the practice of orthopedic surgery. AAOS, Chicago, 1989.

29. Klein RS, Phelan JA, Freeman K *et al.* Low occupational health risk of human immunodeficiency virus infection amongst dental professionals. *N Eng J Med* 1988; **318**:86–90.

30. Garden JM *et al.* Papillomavirus in the vapor of carbon dioxide laser-treated verrucae. *JAMA* 1988; **259**:1199–202.

31. Ferenczy A, Bergeron C, Richart RM. Human papillomavirus DNA in CO_2 laser-generated plume of smoke and its consequences to the surgeon. *Obstet Gynecol* 1990; **75**:114–18.

32. British Medical Association. A code of practice for the safe use and disposal of sharps. BMA, London, 1990.

33. Henderson DK, Gerberding JL. Prophylactic zidovudine after occupational exposure to the human immunodeficiency virus: an interim analysis. *J Infect Dis* 1989; **160**:321–7.

34. Centers for Disease Control. Public Health Service statement on management of occupational exposure to HIV, including considerations regarding zidovudine postexposure use. *MMWR* 1990; **39**:RR-1.

35. Sacho H, Schoub BD. Guidelines for the use of zidovudine for post-exposure prophylaxis after needlestick injuries in health care settings. *S Afr Med J* 1990; **77**:619–22.

36. Sacks HS, Rose DN. Zidovudine prophylaxis for needlestick exposure to human immunodeficiency virus: a decision analysis. *J Gen Intern Med* 1990; **5**:132–7.

37. Zidovudine and needlestick exposure. *Lancet* 1990; **335**:1271.
38. Morgan DR. HIV and needlestick injuries. *Lancet* 1990; **335**:1280.
39. Ryhanen P, Jouppila R, Lanning M *et al*. Natural killer cell activity after elective caesarean section under general anaesthesia and epidural anaesthesia in healthy parturients and their newborn. *Gynaecol Obstet Invest* 1985; **19**:139–42.
40. Konotey-Ahulu FID. Surgery and the risk of AIDS in HIV-positive patients. *Lancet* 1987; **2**:1146.

5

Protection of the surgeon
John Rainey

Introduction

Despite continuing progress and advances in the practice of surgery, infection remains foremost of the many risks which attend a surgical operation. Infection is also unique among surgical hazards in that the surgeon and his team, may, on occasion, be as vulnerable to it as the patient.

Prevention of transmission of infection between surgeon and patient in either direction depends on the creation and maintenance of a barrier between the tissues of the patient and those of the surgeon, assistants and all paramedical staff.

Prior to the introduction of Lister's principles of antisepsis in 1867 with dramatic improvements in postoperative infection rates, surgeons paid scant attention to the concept of maintaining a physical or chemical barrier between themselves and their patients. Frock coats, donned before an operating session, and worn throughout, merely served to protect their everyday clothes. They became stiffened and crusted with pus, blood and other debris and were rarely, if ever, cleaned. Hands were not gloved, and before Semmelweiss (1847) were washed only when necessary to remove unpleasant and smelly substances.

The era of antisepsis, developed for the protection of the patient, gradually evolved into the era of aseptic surgery with the introduction of techniques for the sterilization of instruments and drapes. Cleaned scrub suits replaced outdoor clothes and surgeons routinely donned caps, masks and sterile gloves and gowns. As individual surgical specialities emerged, each designed complex rituals to solve their own particular infection control problems and to enhance further the sterility of the operative field. Determined at all costs to keep micro-organisms away from the patient, orthopedic surgeons pioneered correct design of theatre ventilation, the use of sterile chambers and laminar flow apparatus, and were the first to adopt double-gloving as routine practice. Gastrointestinal surgeons, by contrast, operating often in an already infected area, were more concerned with minimizing rather than eliminating exposure of the patient to potential pathogens, employing special draping systems, closed anastomoses and non-touch techniques.

Maintenance of correct aseptic technique was particularly crucial in surgical practice before the advent of antibiotics. These agents, used therapeutically and especially prophylactically, have clearly had a major impact of the incidence and consequence of postoperative infection in many fields. As a result, strict and obsessive adherence to aseptic principles might, for a time, have been considered less important than in pre-antibiotic days. However, as the threat of significant bacterial infection has receded it has been replaced by that of the more insidious viral pathogens; hepatitis B virus (HBV) was initially the most dreaded following outbreaks among immunosuppressed patients in renal dialysis and transplant units during the late 1960s. More recently, HIV infection has understandably become the most prominent virus in this context.

While most surgical infection results from contamination of exposed and unprotected tissues by bacteria from the patient's own flora, the environment or the surgeon's skin or mucous membranes, these viral pathogens are transmitted by the blood-borne route. This can only occur when there is direct contact between the blood and/or tissues of the patient and those of the surgeon, a situation which allows the possibility of transmission of infection in either direction. An obvious example is needlestick injury in which the needle, having passed through the tissues of the operative field, then pierces the surgeon's glove and his skin.

In fact, surgical staff seem to be more at risk from these viruses than do their patients. In 1986, the Hepatitis Epidemiology Unit estimated that the average annual risk, in the UK, of HBV infection being transmitted to patients by carriers of hepatitis B surface antigen (HBsAg) involved in invasive surgical procedures was one in one million operations, whereas the estimation of risk of infection being tramsmitted from patient to surgeon was 25 per 100 000 [1]. Furthermore, while approximately 30 health-care workers worldwide have become HIV positive following contact with infected patients, there is, as yet, no reported case of a patient being infected with HIV following contact with hospital staff in the course of their duties [2].

Risks in routine surgery

Surgeons are now faced with the disturbing possibility that taking part in a surgical operation may in some cases be more hazardous for them than for the patient. Ever since John Hunter deliberately inoculated himself with syphilis (1767), with unforeseen and ultimately tragic results, surgeons have been aware of the particular danger of working with sharp instruments in potentially infected tissues. At the turn of this century, a leading London surgeon committed suicide on discovering that he had infected his wife with syphilis which had been acquired as a result of a cut sustained while operating on an infected patient. As recently as the Second World War, cases were recorded of surgeons developing syphilitic lesions in such circumstances [3]. Perhaps the most prominent survivor of serious soft tissue infection acquired while operating was Hamilton Bailey (1894–61) who lost the index finger of his left hand (as can be seen in many photographs in the earlier editions of his textbooks).

The understandable concern among surgical staff about the risk of acquiring acute hepatitis B (AHB) from suspected or unsuspected carriers has been somewhat allayed by the development of effective and safe immunization [4]. By contrast, worries about the rising incidence of HIV infection not only in recognized risk groups, but also more stealthily among the general heterosexual population [5], have not been offset by any such comforting developments. The first deaths among doctors and other health-care workers from AIDS acquired at work focused the attention of the medical community on the risks of HIV infection transmitted from known or unknown patient carriers to those caring for them. As a result, some groups have pressed for routine testing for HIV for all patients entering hospital, or at least for all patients from recognized high-risk groups scheduled for surgery. On the other hand, intensive media coverage has suggested to the public that they could also be vulnerable to HIV infection passed in the opposite direction, leading to demands for HIV testing of all surgeons and staff involved in surgery. Since, for a number of reasons, neither of these Draconian measures seems likely to be introduced, it is appropriate to review current surgical practice in the light of scanty and incomplete knowledge of the incidence of HIV infection in the general population.

While it is HIV that causes most concern, it should be remembered that HBV is much more infectious and is frequently encountered in the same risk groups and indeed in the same patients, and that the available data suggest that its incidence continues to increase [4,6]. Furthermore, both cytomegalovirus and herpes simplex virus can be transmitted in similar fashion.

In contrast to the situation for HIV, the risks and consequence of hospital-acquired AHB for both patients and staff have been fairly well defined and documented [1].

The risk of subsequent development of AHB in hospital staff may be as high as 35% after a single needlestick injury sustained during surgery on a high-risk antigen carrier [7]. Although the risk of developing AHB after such an incident may be reduced significantly by the administration of anti-hepatitis immunoglobulin [8], and 90–95% of those infected become seronegative within one year, there is an appreciable mortality for the disease of up to 2% in older patients [9], and some are left with a legacy of chronic persistent or chronic active hepatitis, cirrhosis or hepatocellular cancer [4].

The potential risk of transmission of HBV infection from medical staff to patients has been confirmed in many studies. Outbreaks or clusters of HBV infection among patients have been traced back to carriers of hepatitis B surface antigen who have been involved in invasive surgical procedures, usually within the previous six months [1,10].

Athough AHB remains a relatively uncommon disease in the UK, the incidence and risks of acquiring this infection for both patients and staff could be reduced with the application of appropriate measures such as screening and immunization, and with improved procedures and techniques in theater.

While there may be a case for screening all hospital admissions for carriers of HBsAg—supported by the 0.1% estimated carrier rate in the normal population [4]—it would seem undeniably prudent to screen at least those patients known to be in high-risk categories. Once the patient has been identified as an HBsAg carrier appropriate safety measures can be taken.

Although the chances of a patient becoming infected by the surgical personnel during an operation may be small, there may still be an argument for routine screening of all staff at the start of their employment and at regular intervals thereafter. A carrier rate of 0.6% was reported from screening 500 UK dentists and there is no reason to assume that the figure for surgeons would be lower [10]. Many units, particularly those treating immunosuppressed patients, already insist on testing all staff for HBsAg.

Among staff carriers, it appears that only those who are actively involved in invasive operations, where sharp instruments and needles are employed, constitute a hazard to patients. In a US study, 228 known inpatient contacts of five proven health-care worker carriers were followed up prospectively for 6–9 months [11]. None of the carriers was involved in invasive procedures on patients and none of the patients developed either clinical or immunological evidence of HBV infection.

A surgeon found to be HBsAg or HBeAg positive should be restricted to clinical duties and prevented from taking part in any invasive procedures. In most cases, of course, he or she will become seronegative within a year and will be able to return safely to normal work.

With the recent development of safe and effective immunization against HBV, the emphasis should change towards prevention of infection: all staff should be immunized at the beginning of their employment [4]. There is also the possibility of extending such a program to encompass high-risk groups, though compliance and follow-up may prove to be difficult.

Needlestick injuries, which occur in up to 1 in 20 operations and are usually sustained by the surgeon, must clearly be considered to constitute the main danger of transmission of HIV infection [12,13]. This is discussed in detail in Chapter 4.

Attempts to reduce the risks to patients and hospital staff of acquiring such infection during professional encounters are bedeviled by the lack of accurate figures on the true incidence of AIDS or HIV infection in the general population. Even if practical or ethical objections to universal screening were overcome, its introduction might not be particularly helpful because of the invariably lengthy lag time between infection and presumed infectivity and seroconversion [14].

Consequently, hospital staff can only attempt to identify high-risk patients and to adopt similar ward and theater procedures to those practiced in known cases of HBV positivity, as described in Chapter 4. However, growing unease about the increasing prevalence of unsuspected HIV infection in the apparently 'normal' heterosexual population suggests that the exercise of classifying patients as high or low risk cannot be reliable and surgeons must inevitably come to assume that all patients *may* be harboring HIV. This heightened awareness of risk should stimulate penetrating questioning and review of current routine procedures in surgical practice.

Most of the data on risk of transmission of HIV infection refer to exposure to infected blood. The virus can, however, be identified in the patient's tissues and body fluids and particularly in semen, plasma, breast milk, CSF and tears [15]. All organs are potentially infectious. Therefore, in addition to avoiding injury with contaminated sharp instruments, staff should avoid unprotected contact with bodily secretions, taking particular care to avoid the contamination of cuts, cracked or broken skin, mucous membranes of the mouth and nose and the eye.

For the surgeon who has the misfortune to become HIV positive, there is little hope of ever becoming seronegative. The Expert Advisory Group on AIDS, while accepting that the risk of a doctor infecting a patient is extremely slight, has made several recommendations on the steps to be taken in such cases [16]. In particular:

'Health Care Workers who consider that they may have been infected with HIV should seek immediate counselling and, if appropriate, diagnostic HIV testing. If found to be infected and if their duties involve performing or assisting in surgical or invasive procedures, they must seek and act upon occupational advice on any modifications or limitations to their duties which may be necessary for the protection of patients.'

In short, a surgeon who is HIV positive would have to give up operating; probably forever. If he refused to do so, he could be reported to the General Medical Council who would have the power to compel him to comply. Furthermore, a surgeon who continues to operate knowing that he may be infectious lays himself open to litigation should a patient subsequently develop HIV infection.

Areas of concern in current practice

Surgeons will have to accept that they have a major responsibility adequately to protect themselves and their staff from potentially dangerous contamination of unexpectedly infectious tissues or body fluids. This objective can be achieved mainly by staff education and a general tightening up of hospital and particularly theater procedures to eliminate the sort of sloppy habits which can be seen in many surgical theaters at present.

A lay observer might well be surprised at the way in which surgical staff (medical and nursing) expose themselves, often, unwittingly, though sometimes carelessly, to the risk of infection. At the start of an operation, a hurriedly made, imprecise and roughly handled incision can cause blood to spurt from several vessels simultaneously into the faces and particularly the eyes of the operating team. Those who normally wear spectacles are often surprised to see just how much blood has splashed on to them by the end of a seemingly straightforward procedure (Fig. 5.1).

Towards the end of many laparotomies, copious saline or antibiotic lavage is necessary. The lavage fluid often spills over the edges of the wound, soaking the drapes; these are usually not waterproof and in turn soak the surgeon's and assistant's gowns (Fig. 5.2) and often their scrub suits and underwear (Fig. 5.3). It is reasonable to speculate that having one's genitals liberally washed in potentially infected fluid cannot be considered safe, whether or not it is diluted with saline or antibiotics.

Furthermore, the part of the sleeve immediately proximal to the glove is often thoroughly soaked, so that, when the gown is eventually stripped off, the wrists are wet and blood-stained (Fig. 5.4).

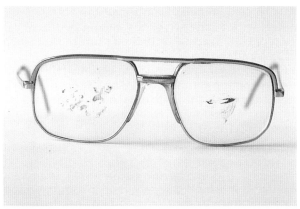

Figure 5.1   Evidence of blood splashed on to a surgeon's spectacles during a 'routine' operation.

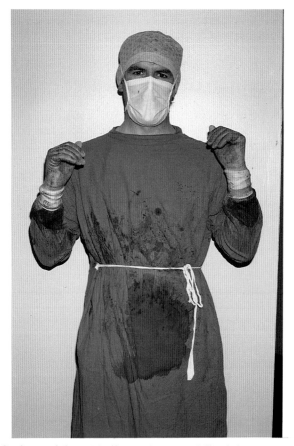

Figure 5.2   Soakage of the midriff area during a difficult laparotomy.

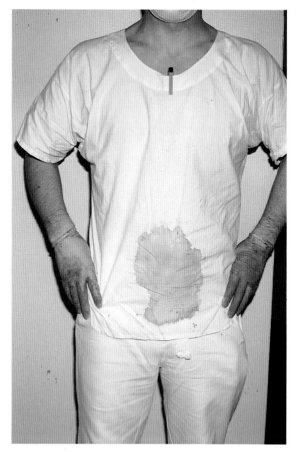

Figure 5.3   Soakage through to the scrub suit and underwear.

When disposable, non-absorbent drapes are (inappropriately) used, considerable amounts of blood and fluid run on to the surgeon's footwear, which can become heavily splattered with blood. The combination of non-absorbent drapes and standard hospital gowns is particularly uncomfortable for the wearers.

The hands are, of course, the areas most vulnerable to hazardous contamination, despite being routinely protected by surgical gloves. These provide a barrier against the micro-organisms of both the surgeon and the patient, and the risk of one infecting the other is virtually eliminated as long as the barrier remains intact. However, gloves offer little protection against needlestick injuries occurring in up to 5% of general surgical operations [12]. These painful incidents often occur towards the end of operations during wound closure when attention may wander and the procedure become 'casual'. The tendency to use fingers as forceps during mass closure with large cutting needles seems particularly dangerous.

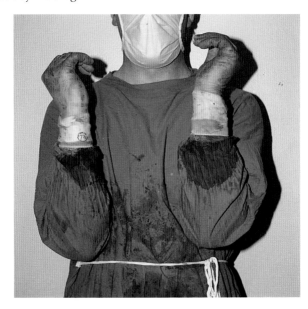

Figure 5.4   Sodden wrists above cuffs and gloves.

In addition, there is an even greater risk of glove perforation without damage to the wearer's skin ranging from 11% to 38% in general surgery [17–19]. This problem may also occur in up to 40% of cardiac operations [20,21] and has been documented in many other fields including cardiac catheterization and oral and dental surgery [22,23]. In more than 50% of these cases, the wearer becomes aware of the damage only when the glove has been removed, revealing a soggy, wet finger (Figs 5.5 an 5.6). As in the case of needlestick injuries, in right-handed individuals the left glove is most often damaged, the index finger and first web space being the commonest

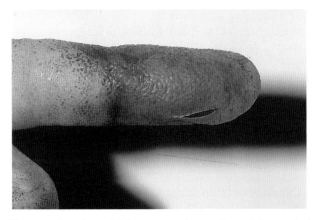

Figure 5.5   Glove perforation which went undetected until the end of a procedure (and see Fig. 5.6).

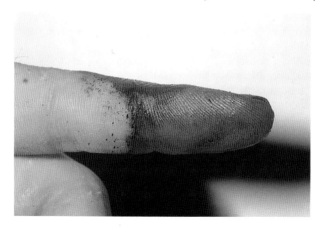

Figure 5.6 Soggy finger (left index) after the glove in Fig. 5.5 had been removed.

sites (Fig. 5.7). This type of contamination poses no obvious threat provided that the skin is intact. Unfortunately the skin of a surgeon's hands is by no means always intact. Surgeons often enjoy hobbies which involve using their hands, such as DIY and gardening, and these commonly result in cuts and abrasions to skin which has been softened by repeated washing and regular prolonged encarceration in rubber gloves. Even a gentle round of golf may cause blisters and cracks in such vulnerable tissue. HIV has been transmitted via infected blood seeping through gauze onto the draped un-gloved hands of a nurse [24].

Ancillary staff, not part of the operating team, may also be exposed to risk unnecessarily. At the end of an operation it is common to see the floor nurses and even auxilliary nurses being helpful by rapidly removing the drapes from a patient, perhaps to allow the anesthetist access to the airway or to facilitate the application of the wound dressing. These individuals,

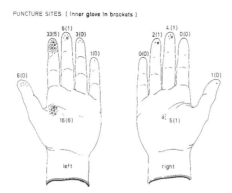

Figure 5.7 Frequency and sites of glove perforation from a study of double-gloving; circles, and the numbers in brackets, indicate where both outer and inner gloves were perforated in this right-hand individual.

who rarely wear gloves, may be expected to pick up discarded surgical gowns and other material carelessly dropped by more 'responsible' members of the operating team.

While detailed protocols for the sterilization of endoscopes have been introduced widely, little attention has been paid to the safety aspect of handling the instruments themselves during and between procedures. The endoscopist's eyes, nose and mouth are often uncomfortably close to the patient and well placed to be sprayed by various aerosols of blood and gastrointestinal secretions, blowing back from faulty valves or imperfectly sealed instrument channels. Therapeutic endoscopy, in particular, may pose problems if long, flexible and often blood-smeared cannulas and guidewires are inadequately controlled.

Protection for staff

In practice most of the problems outlined above should be largely solved, and the dangers of theater work for all concerned appreciably reduced, by education of all staff and a general improvement in operating theater routines, essentially returning to the principles of aseptic surgery and the maintenance of an intact barrier between surgeon and patient.

Gloves

Surgical gloves are the key elements in the protection of staff and patients alike. The introduction of rubber gloves in surgical operations is usually attributed to WS Halsted of the Johns Hopkins Hospital, Baltimore, in 1899/90 [25]. He was initially concerned simply to protect his scrub nurse's hands from dermatitis induced by mercuric chloride. Strangely, he did not report his experience with surgical gloving until 1913 [26] while his colleague at the same institution, HH Robb, a gynecologist, published a book on 'aseptic surgical technique' in 1894 in which operators were recommended to wear gloves routinely. Halstead's assistant, Joseph Bloodgood, may have been the first to recognize the potential benefits for patients when he reported objective evidence that hernia wound infection rates were very much reduced when gloves were worn [27]. Interestingly, none of the surgeons of this period wore gowns.

Claims have been made for several European surgeons as the instigators of surgical gloving at around that period [28]. However, the surgical use of gloves had in fact been advocated more than a century before. In 1758, JJ Walbaum devised an obstetric 'glove' made from the cecum of a sheep; and in 1834, RF Cook stated with almost unbelievable foresight that 'a pair of India rubber gloves would be perfectly impenetratable to the most malignant virus'. Perhaps the real credit for the invention of surgical rubber gloves should go to Charles Goodyear who initiated the research that led to the vulcanization of rubber in the early 1840s, making possible the subsequent manufacture of these essential accessories to surgical practice [29].

Some conservative surgeons felt that gloves were more a hindrance than a help in the operative field, but their doubts were gradually overcome and by

1910 gloves were almost universally accepted. A few eminent surgeons continued to remove their gloves during particularly delicate phases of some operations until the 1960s [25].

Today there is little debate about the necessity for donning gloves when involved in invasive procedures of any kind. This practice should extend routinely to all who may potentially be in contact with infective material. This means that not only surgeons, but also anesthetists, casualty staff, radiologists and many other specialists should use this form of hand protection. Nurses, particularly those in intensive therapy units, should be gloved during procedures such as sucking out and clearing endotracheal and tracheostomy tubes, and when carrying out many aspects of routine nursing care such as dressing changes and the adjustment of intravenous and intra-arterial lines [30]. In addition, mortuary and autopsy room staff and those working in all laboratories handling human tissue are increasingly being encouraged to wear gloves. Such protection should be provided for hospital domestic staff, particularly those cleaning theaters and dealing with soiled floors and carpets.

Patients and their relatives may initially find routine wearing of gloves by more and more hospital staff somewhat threatening [31] but may be reassured by the knowledge that such measures contribute greatly to overall infection control and significantly decrease the incidence of many different types of hospital-acquired infections among staff and patients alike [32,33].

A number of further measures could improve the protective effectiveness of surgeons' gloves. Double-gloving should perhaps be recommended for all operations: this already applies in many orthopedic units [34]. Wearing two pairs of gloves appears to reduce significantly the incidence of hand or finger contamination, by maintaining a barrier (the inner glove) between the wearer and patient in four out of five cases where the outer glove has been breached (Fig. 5.7).

Initially, acceptance of double-gloving may be difficult because of discomfort. Sometimes this is reduced by having the inner glove half a size *larger* than the outer, following the principle of the tailor who uses more material for the lining of the sleeve than for the sleeve itself. Surgical staff will have to weigh the enhanced safety of introducing a second barrier between themselves and the patient against possible discomfort or reduced sensitivity and dexterity.

Whether double or single gloves are to be used, those lined with a hydrogel rather than with corn starch may be more appropriate since these are easily donned, and have a biocompatible lining. Hydrogels appear to inhibit bacterial regrowth and may also have some antiviral properties [35].

It is interesting to read that Halstead's original requirement for gloves was that they should have gauntlets to protect the wrists [25]. This idea could perhaps be reintroduced in the form of gloves with longer reinforced cuffs extending well up the forearm to prevent soakage of the gown sleeve.

Double-gloving, of course, offers little or no protection against the carelessly wielded knife or needle. The advent of gloves sufficiently strong to deflect a blade or needle point is eagerly awaited. In the meantime, a *thimble* worn between two sets of gloves, to protect the distal part of the index finger, has been suggested to improve protection when operating on high-risk cases [36]. Another idea has been to bind the distal phalanges where possible with several layers of adhesive tape prior to donning gloves [37].

Closer attention to surgical technique could reduce the incidence of needlestick injuries to less than 3% [6]. For example, trainees must be discouraged from substituting fingers for forceps during dissection or suturing. Needles and sharp instruments should be routinely handled in the same careful way as described for high-risk patients. In the future, knives may ultimately be replaced by alternative and less dangerous instruments, such as diathermy or laser knives; very little blood is spilled when these instruments are used and there is little risk of needlestick injury. The use of staples to replace sutures for gastrointestinal anastomoses and skin closure, debatable on grounds of cost, should perhaps be encouraged for reasons of safety.

Gowns and drapes

Reusable woven fabrics, such as cotton, have been universally used as aseptic gowns and drapes since the turn of the century. Such fabrics are readily obtainable, easy to work with and comfortable to wear and were originally thought to provide an acceptable barrier. This last and most essential requirement was held to be true until 1952 when Beck demonstrated that, although woven materials were effective when dry, they became totally porous to micro-organisms when wet, however many layers were used [38].

Since then a great deal of research has been deployed to develop appropriate materials, either disposable or reusable, which are resistent to aqueous penetration. Many such materials have emerged over the years but as yet none has gained general acceptance or succeeded in displacing standard woven fabrics from routine use in operative surgery. Clearly any new material must be shown to be an effective barrier to organisms when wet since its primary role is to maintain aseptic technique and to reduce or prevent surgical sepsis. There are conflicting reports of the success of several non-woven materials in this respect [39,40]. A recent unpublished survey of synthetic disposable and reusable gowns available in the author's Health Board Area revealed that, within 60 minutes, saline had seeped through all the materials tested. Although less permeable to aqueous solutions than cotton, none of the gowns could be considered completely impermeable. In 1988, the Association of Operating Room Nurses in the USA, recognizing the need for innovation in this area, published Recommended Practices for the development and evaluation of materials for surgical gowns and drapes [41]. In addition to the basic barrier qualities outlined above, they pointed out that gowns should allow freedom of movement and prevent excessive heat build-up. Drapes should conform to body contours and maintain an isothermic environment appropriate to body temperature.

In the study referred to above, several practical problems emerged with all types of disposable drapes. Users commented that they were acceptable for abdominal procedures performed over a relatively flat area when they were easily laid on and secured with adhesive strips. However, it proved more difficult to drape limbs and the head, where the material did not conform well, tending to slip, particularly during long procedures and when some repositioning of the operative site was required. The necessity of achieving complete drying of the skin prior to the application of drapes was considered tiresome and some patients developed skin reactions to the adhesive strips. In general, the more expensive reusable drapes performed more satis-factorily especially when used with specifically designed atraumatic towel clips.

A less obvious but relevant safety issue concerns the flammability proper-ties of gown and drape materials, particularly in the light of increasing use of lasers and other high-energy devices. The fiber content of such materials may also be important. Some non-woven disposable materials contain cellulose (wood pulp) fibers which are released into the atmosphere on mild abrasion and which may be associated with postoperative complications such as keloid scars, wound dehiscence and incisional hernias [42,43]. In addition, any material must be free of toxic ingredients particularly in drapes where there will be direct skin or open-wound contact. In the absence of a widely available gown and drape material which meets all these stringent criteria and which is cost-effective, surgeons may still have to rely on simple reusable woven cotton, despite its known deficiency as a barrier in routine surgery. Wearing a plastic apron beneath the gown for added protection against 'soak-through' might seem sensible but is unlikely to gain wide-spread acceptance because of the extremely uncomfortable overheating and excessive sweating beneath it. Small disposable adhesive plastic aprons applied to the midriff after gowning may be the most reasonable compromise.

Masks

While the wearing of gowns and gloves is mandatory in surgery, the case for donning face masks can be challenged on bacteriological grounds. This largely academic controversy has been overshadowed by the need for routine safety precautions in theater. Masks must be worn by all the operating team since they cover the nose and mouth and protect mucous membranes from accidental splashes.

Glasses and goggles

The eyes should also be protected at all times. Those who wear glasses should continue to do so and not succumb to the vanity—or indeed folly—of contact lenses, at least in theater. Those with good eyesight might consider having plain glasses fitted as these are generally more comfortable than any type of goggles currently available and are almost as effective.

Economic considerations

Clearly, the process of improving safety standards in surgery has major economic implications. Routine operations may take longer, and theater (and consequently bed) throughput rates may decrease to a variable degree, resulting in reduced efficiency.

Generally increased glove usage throughout hospitals may stretch already tight budgets. In the author's own general hospital serving a population of 150 000, in which 14 000 operations are carried out annually, expenditure on gloves rose by £20 000 or 35% in one year (1988/89). This increase predates the introduction of double-gloving which is not, as yet, routine practice. No specific funds have been identified to cover these costs which will have to be met from the general unit budget.

Although all those who need protection must be adequately supplied, it is important to ensure that the type of gloves provided are appropriate for the area of hospital practice in which they are to be used [44]. Surgeons may need expensive hydrogel-lined, sensitive sterile gloves, but those worn by laboratory technicians can be cheaper, less sensitive and non-sterile. Gloves for internal examinations in outpatient clinics are of even lower specification. Staff should be trained to don and remove gloves safely [45], and in many clinical situations it is acceptable and safe to wash surgical gloves with standard antiseptic preparation prior to reusing them [46,47].

The cost implications of switching to more effective barrier materials for drapes and gowns are more difficult to define. The sparse published data on the question are inconclusive. Most of the cost information available is being disseminated by companies with vested commercial interests [48].

The long-term economics of reusable materials have to be compared with the short-term expense of disposables. Associated factors must also be taken into account such as the cost, availability and accessability of laundering facilities versus storage space, delivery capability and cost of disposal for disposables. A recent cost–benefit analysis of various materials for drapes and gowns in the author's own hospital produced only one firm conclusion: any change from the status quo (cotton) would involve increased expenditure in both the short term and the long term, and therefore, in the current financial climate, would be out of the question.

Nevertheless, since most hospitals are now obliged to carry stocks of disposable gowns and drapes, for use in recognized high-risk cases, surgeons are well placed to evaluate the various available products and to identify those which come closest to meeting their surgical and safety criteria.

Summary

While the techniques and precautions for operations on high-risk patients are well-established, constantly refined and updated, there is scope for considerable improvement in routine operating theater procedures. The aim must be to eliminate (or at least keep to a minimum) the chances of staff succumbing to potentially disastrous occupational hazards such as infection with HBV or HIV. Heightened awareness of risk and increased safety consciousness in surgical practice should go some way to achieving this objective and to avoiding the worst possible scenario: that of a non-infected patient acquiring such infection during the course of surgical treatment.

References

1. Polakoff S. Acute hepatitis B in patients in Britain related to previous operations and dental treatment. *BMJ* 1986; 293:33–6.
2. Wastell C. Aids and the surgeon: an update. In *Risks and Complications: The Patient and Surgeon in Theatre.* Oxford: Medicine Group (UK) Ltd, 1989: 9–10.
3. Fraser I. *Blood, Sweat and Cheers.* Cambridge: Cambridge University Press, 1989.
4. Finch RG. Time for action on hepatitis B immunisation. *BMJ* 1987; 294: 197–8.
5. AIDS: Scotland. An epidemiological update on AIDS and HIV for the GP in Scotland. Communicable Diseases (Scotland) Unit in collaboration with the Scottish Home and Health Department. Issue 5; 1990.
6. Johnson CD, Evans R, Shanson DC, Wastell C. Attitudes of operating theatre staff to inoculation-risk cases. *Br J Surg* 1989; 76:195–7.
7. Bradbeer C. AIDS—epidemiology and screening. *Med Internat* 1986; 2:1241–6.
8. A combined Medical Research Council and Public Health Laboratory Service Report: The incidence of hepatitis B infection after accidental exposure and anti-HBV immunoglobulin phophylasis. *Lancet* 1980; i:6–8.
9. Polakoff S. Acute viral hepatitis B: laboratory reports 1980–84. *BMJ* 1986; 293:37–8.
10. Report of a collaborative study by the Communicable Disease Surveillance Centre and the Epidemiological Research Laboratory of the Public Health Laboratory Service together with a District Control-of-Infection Service: Acute hepatitis B associated with gynaecological surgery. *Lancet* 1980; i:1–6.
11. Alter HJ, Chalmers TC, Freeman BM, *et al.* Wealth-care workers positive for hepatitis B surface antigen: Are their contacts at risk? *New Engl J Med* 1975; 292 (9):454–7.
12. Hassain SA, Latif ABA, Choudhary AAAA. Risk to surgeons: a survey of accidental injuries during operations. *Br J Surg* 1988; 75:314–16.
13. Dudley HAF, Sim A. AIDS: a bill of rights for the surgical team? *BMJ* 1988; 296:1449–50.
14. McEwen LM. Guidelines in HIV infection, *BMJ* 1989; 299:182.
15. Forbes CD. The surgeon and HTLV-III infection. *Br J Surg* 1986; 73: 168–9.
16. Department of Health and Social Security. AIDS/HIV infected health care workers. *London*: DHSS, 1988.
17. Matta H, Thompson AM, Rainey JB. Does wearing two pairs of gloves protect operating theatre staff from skin contamination? *BMJ* 1988; 297:597–8.
18. Dodds RDA, Guy PJ, Peacock AM, Duffy SR, Barker SGE, Thomas MH. Surgical glove perforation. *Br J Surg* 1988; 75:966–8.
19. Brough SJ, Hunt TM, Barrie WW. Surgical glove perforations. *Br J Surg* 1988; 75:317–18.
20. Berg GA, Kirk AJB, Bain WH. Punctured surgical gloves and bacterial recolonisation of hands during open heart surgery: implications for prosthetic valve replacement. *Br J Clin Pract* 1987; 41:903–6.
21. Hosie KB, Dunning JJ, Bailey JS, Firmin RK. Glove perforation during sternotomy closure. *Lancet* 1988; ii:1500.
22. Palmisano JM, Meliones JN. Damage to physicians gloves during routine cardiac catheterisation: an underappreciated occurrence. *J Am Coll Cardiol* 1989; 14:(96): 1527–9.
23. Jakush J. Infection control in the dental office: a realistic approach. *JADA* 1986; 112:459–68.
24. Ezzell C. Hospital workers have AIDS virus. *Nature* 1987; 327:261.
25. Geelhoed GW. The pre-Halstedian and post-Halstedian history of the surgical rubber glove. *Surg Gynaecol Obstet* 1988; 167:350–6.

26. Halsted WS. Ligature and suture material. *JAMA* 1913; **60**:1119–26.
27. Walter CW. Use of surgical rubber gloves. *Surgery* 1983; **93** (5):728.
28. Miller JM. William Stewart Halstead and the use of the surgical rubber glove. *Surgery* 1982; **92**:541–3.
29. Williams TG. History of theatre rituals—safer surgery. In *Risks and Complications: The Patient and Surgeon in Theatre*. Oxford: Medicine Group (UK) Ltd, 1989: 3.
30. Williams DK. Two-glove technique. *Focus Crit Care* 1988; **15**:8.
31. Siegel LJ, Smith KE. Infection control barrier techniques used by physicians during routine examinations—parental attitudes. *Clin Paediatrics* 1989; **28**:231–4.
32. Leclair JM, Freeman J. Sullivan BF, Crowley CM, Goldman DA. Prevention of nosocomial respiratory syncytial virus infections through compliance with glove and gown isolation precautions. *New Engl J Med* 1987; **317**:329–34.
33. Johnson S, Gerding DM, Olson MM, *et al*. Prospective controlled study of vinyl glove use to interrupt *Clostridium difficile* nosocomial transmission. *Am. J Med* 1990; **88**:137–40.
34. McCue SF, Berg, EW, Saunders EA. Efficiency of double-gloving as a barrier to microbial contamination during total joint arthroplasty. *J Bone Joint Surg* 1981; **63**:811–3.
35. Dalgleish AG, Malkovsky M. Surgical gloves as a mechanical barrier against human immuno-deficiency viruses. *Br J Surg* 1988; **75**:171–2.
36. Miles AJG, Wastell C, Allen-Mersh TG. Protection for the left index finger whilst operating on HIV positive patients. *Ann R Coll Surg Engl* 1989; **71**:225.
37. Paglia SL, Sommer RM. AIDS infection protection—reinforced gloves. *Anesth Analg* 1989; **69**:407.
38. Beck WC, Collette TA. False faiths in the surgeon's gown and surgical drape. *Am J Surg* 1952; **83**:125–6.
39 Moylan JA, Fitzpatrick KT, Davenport KE. Reducing wound infections. *Arch Surg* 1987; **122**:152–7.
40. Garibaldi RA, Maglio S, Lerer T, *et al*. Comparison of non-woven and woven gown and drape fabric to prevent intraoperative wound contamination and postoperative infection. *Am J Surg* 1986; **152**:505–9.
41. AORN Recommended Practices Subcommittee. Recommended practices—aseptic barrier materials for surgical gowns and drapes. *AORN J* 1988; **47**:572–6.
42. Tucker M, Burdman D, Deysime M, *et al*. Granulomatous peritonitis due to cellular fibers from disposable surgical fabrics. *Am Surg* 1974; **180**:831–5.
43. Dragan MJ. Wood fibres from disposable surgical gowns and drapes. *JAMA* 1979; **241**:2297–8.
44. Standring JA. Disposable gloves: a study of the uses, relative advantages and cost of disposable gloves. *Nursing Times* 1980; **34** (Suppl. 14): 15–18.
45. The rights and wrongs of rubber gloves. *Occupational Health* 1987; **39**:58–9.
46. Doebbeling BN, Pfaller MD, Houston AK, Weuzel RP. Removal of nosocomial pathogens from the contaminated glove: implications for glove reuse and handwashing. *Ann Intern Med* 1988; **109**:394–8.
47. Douglas CWI, Millwood TA, Clark A. The use of various handwashing agents to decontaminate gloved hands. *Br Dent J* 1989; **167**:62–5.
48. Belkin NL. Surgical gowns and drapes as aseptic barriers. *Am J Infect Control* 1988; **16**:14–18.

6

Examination of the anus and rectum in the HIV infected patient
William P Schecter

HIV infection is a spectrum of disease ranging from the asymptomatic infected patient to the patient with advanced AIDS. HIV infected patients can present with anorectal complaints caused by conditions either (1) unrelated to their infection, (2) associated with anal intercourse, or (3) caused by neoplasia or opportunistic infection specifically related to AIDS. The possibility of HIV infection should be considered in all patients with anorectal complaints.

History taking

Patients usually present with one or more of the following complaints: (1) pain, (2) bleeding, (3) drainage, (4) diarrhea, (5) a mass, or (6) incontinence. The duration and frequency of the specific complaint should be noted as well as any measures which relieve the symptoms. The frequency, consistency, caliber and color of bowel movements, as well as any change in bowel habits, may provide important diagnostic clues. A dietary history, particularly for constipated patients, is extremely important. Information regarding the type of undergarments, laundry soaps and the use of fragrances and creams is useful in the evaluation of patients complaining of pruritis ani.

A careful history regarding anal intercourse is important in the evaluation of anorectal complaints and in identifying patients at high risk. Questions regarding sexual practices can sometimes be embarrassing for both the doctor and the patient. Inquire in a matter of fact manner whether the patient has pain during anal intercourse: this type of non-judgmental question affords the patient the opportunity to confirm or deny the practice. If the patient is at risk for HIV infection, an HIV test should be recommended. Most of the homosexual men attending the proctology clinic at San Francisco General Hospital have already been tested for HIV antibodies and will so inform the doctor when questioned. A review of 'safer sexual practices' for patients who engage in anal intercourse is an important part of the patient interview [1]. Many homosexual men are well-informed on this subject but the issue should at least be raised. A discussion of 'safer sexual practices' should not be limited to homosexual men. All HIV infected patients can potentially transmit the virus during sexual intercourse. Condoms should always be worn during intercourse [2], but they cannot be considered 100% effective because of the risk of rupture or slippage [3]. Although the possibility of HIV transmission during passionate kissing has been suggested [4], this mode of transmission has not been proven. There is no evidence that social kissing has resulted in HIV transmission [5].

Pain

Proctalgia is the most common presenting complaint of HIV infected patients with anorectal disease. Perianal sepsis, a fissure-in-ano or painful hemorrhoids should be suspected and can be easily diagnosed on physical examination. Occasionally, a patient with an intersphincteric abscess will complain of severe pain and difficulty walking. Inspection of the perianal area may be unrewarding, but a digital examination will be impossible because of pain. Gentle palpation of the perianal area often reveals point tenderness which is an important clue to the location of the abscess. Further evaluation should proceed in the operating theater under anesthesia [6,7].

Patients with more advanced HIV infection may complain of perianal pain caused by more unusual diseases. Perianal herpes simplex and varicella zoster lesions can usually be diagnosed by inspection [8,9]. A few patients with advanced AIDS may have severe pain caused by a solitary ulcer in the anal canal which burrows into the sphincter mechanism [6,10]. Proctitis caused by *Neisseria gonorrhoeae*, Chlamydia, cytomegalovirus, or herpes simplex may cause severe pain [11–13]. Rarely, the pain may be caused by local invasion of the perianal tissues by lymphoma [14], Kaposi's sarcoma [15] or squamous cell carcinoma of the anus [16].

Bleeding

Although anorectal bleeding raises the question of a neoplasm, few HIV infected patients with this complaint have adenocarcinoma of the rectum. The bleeding more often results from fissures, hemorrhoids or coloproctitis. These diseases usually cause multiple symptoms which can be elicited by a careful history. Persistent anorectal bleeding requires a complete evaluation of the colon, rectum and anus to exclude malignancy.

Drainage

The cause of anal discharge in most HIV infected patients is difficult to diagnose. Gonococcal proctitis should be excluded by culture on Thayer–Martin medium. Chlamydial proctitis should be considered. Culture of anal discharge with calcium alginate swabs may reveal chlamydial infection. Alternatively, the patient with persistent unexplained discharge can be given a therapeutic trial with tetracycline or erythromycin.

Mucosal prolapse and a lax anus are commonly associated with discharge. These conditions may be related to prolapsing hemorrhoids [17] or the result of regular receptive anal intercourse. Discharge and soiling are seen most commonly when coloproctitis is present in a patient with a lax anus.

Diarrhea

Persistent diarrhea is a debilitating problem for many patients with advanced AIDS. Coloproctitis may be caused by a variety of opportunistic infections including cytomegalovirus [18], amebiasis [19], cryptosporidiosis [20], and *Mycobacterium avium intracellulare* (MAI) [19]. More commonly, the patient presents with pain due to the irritation of frequent diarrheal bowel movements caused by these infections as well as by Salmonella, Shigella or Campylobacter. Culture of the stool and examination for ova and parasites can sometimes make the diagnosis. Some patients require endoscopic examination of the colon and colorectal biopsies for histology and viral culture. Diarrhea caused by multiple pathogens is the rule rather than the exception.

Perianal mass

Unquestionably the most common cause of a perianal mass in HIV infected patients in our clinic is anal condylomata. Patients with human papillomavirus disease (HPV) are at risk for squamous cell carcinoma of the anus [21], and occasionally an HIV infected patient with anal condylomata will also have an anal squamous cancer [16]. The anal mucosa, like the mucosa of the cervix, can be screened for intraepithelial neoplasia [22]. The precise role of routine screening of patients with anal HPV infection remains to be defined, but a careful evaluation and close follow-up of all patients with anal condylomata is essential.

Other anorectal conditions such as thrombosed hemorrhoids, skin tags and hypertrophied anal papillae may also present as masses. Kaposi's sarcoma (KS) and anorectal lymphoma can occasionally present as a perianal mass in patients with AIDS. The few patients with perianal KS and lymphoma seen by the author already had a diagnosis of AIDS and had advanced disease.

Incontinence

Patients with advanced AIDS may be incontinent for many reasons. Fecal impaction, however, is an unusual cause in this clinical situation. More commonly, diarrhea due to multiple opportunistic infections, inanition and AIDS dementia lead to a loss of control of bowel function [23,24]. Attempts to diagnose and treat diarrhea as well as supportive nursing care are usually only partially successful at correcting the problem [25].

Equipment

The following equipment should be available in the office or clinic for a proper anorectal examination: (1) disposable latex gloves, (2) water-soluble lubricant, (3) 5% xylocaine cream, (4) non-disposable metal anoscopes, (5) rigid sigmoidoscopes, and (6) a selection of biopsy forceps. A selection of fine probes is sometimes helpful for probing fistula tracts. A suction machine can be quite useful.

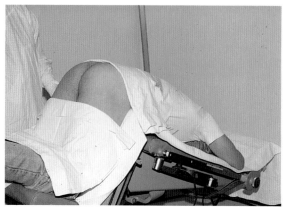

Figure 6.1   Jack-knife (knee-chest) position.

Media for bacteriologic and viral culture should be available. Specimens should be collected and transported using Thayer–Martin medium for *Neisseria gonorrhoeae* and the viral culturette (Becton–Dickinson, Cockeysville, MD, catalog no. 4361514) for viral culture. The physician should indicate which viruses are suspected if viral culture is requested. The Chlamydia transport system should be used for chlamydial culture and the Amies transport medium for routine bacteriologic culture [27].

The author prefers the prone jack-knife position for examination of the anorectum (Fig. 6.1). Our clinic has two examination tables (Fig. 6.2) which tilt the patient head-down, providing access for a complete anorectal exam. Some patients cannot tolerate the prone jack-knife position; these patients are best examined in the left lateral (Sims) position (Fig. 6.3). The patient should be positioned with the buttocks off the examination table supported by a pillow or folded pads. The hips and knees should be flexed as much as possible. If the buttocks are not sufficiently off the table, the examiner's head will hit the table frequently during rigid sigmoidoscopy.

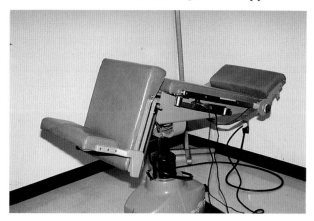

Figure 6.2   Tilting examination table.

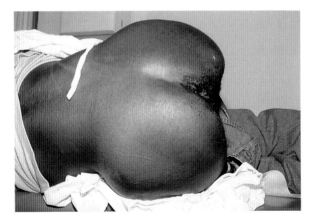

Figure 6.3   Sims position.

Prevention of HIV transmission

The basic principle of universal precautions [26] is that blood and all other body fluids are potentially toxic substances. Contact of patient's blood, stool or secretions which the skin and mucous membranes of the health-care worker is unacceptable. A protective smock, protective eyewear and two pairs of latex gloves should be worn for all examinations. Two pairs of latex gloves should be standard because the failure rate of disposable latex gloves is high [28–30; see also Chapter 5].

DNA from HPV has been recovered from the smoke plume after laser cautery of cutaneous verrucae [31]. If laser or electrocautery is performed in the clinic, masks capable of filtering out particles as small as 0.3 microns and high-power suction devices should be used to evacuate smoke. Although there is no evidence that HIV can be transmitted by inhalation of cautery moke from HIV infected patients, the prudent surgeon will avoid inhaling electrocautery smoke if possible.

Non-disposable metal instruments should be placed immediately in detergent solution after use and gas-sterilized prior to reuse. Disposable plastic instruments should of course be immediately discarded after use. Flip-top garbage bins allow easy access to the bin but preserve the clean appearance and fresh scent of the examination room (Fig. 6.4).

The examination

Spread the buttocks and inspect the skin. Search for the presence of skin lesions which might suggest herpes simplex or zoster infection, fungal infection, fistula-in-ano or perirectal abscess.

Herpes simplex infection appears acutely as painful vesicles containing clear fluid. The vesicles eventually rupture, producing exquisitely tender

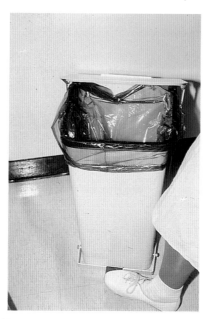

Figure 6.4   Flip-top disposal bin.

superficial moist open sores which usually dry up over a period of several days. Varicella zoster lesions have a similar appearance but tend to cluster in the dermatomal distribution of peripheral nerves. Candida perineal infections appear as moist erythematous rashes with a cheesy white exudate localized to the intertrigenous zones such as the intergluteal fold.

A fistula-in-ano usually presents with a small hole in the perianal region which intermittently drains purulent material. The tissues on either side of the hole are often raised giving the fistula's opening a nipple-like appearance. There is frequently a previous history of a perirectal abscess. The fistula may be associated with anal condylomata (Figs 6.5A and 6.5B). Most fistulae are relatively pain-free unless associated with inadequately drained pus.

A perirectal abscess may be located perianally, between the two anal sphincters, in the ischiorectal fossa or above the levators [32]. Most superficial perirectal abscesses present as obvious exquisitely tender warm erythematous masses. Diagnosis and localization of intersphincteric and supralevator abscesses can be challenging. Examination under anesthesia is required. Identifying the point of maximal perianal tenderness prior to anesthesia is most helpful in localizing the difficult abscess. Rarely, a CT scan may be required to diagnose an occult supralevator abscess.

Search carefully for any evidence of anal fissure, mucosal prolapse or hemorrhoids. An anal fissure is a crack in the mucosa of the anal canal which is found most commonly in the posterior midline. The crack can be extremely painful particularly during defecation. Spread the perianal tissues and ask the patient to bear down. If a fissure is present, it will come into

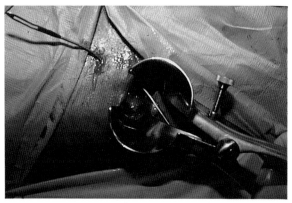

Figure 6.5A Fistual-in-ano.

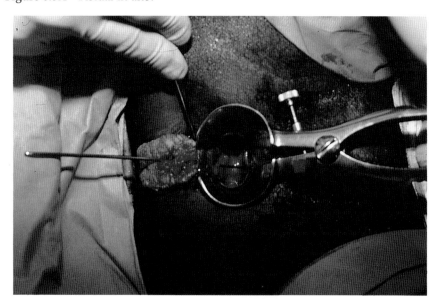

Figure 6.5B Fistual-in-ano associated with anal warts.

view. Mucosal prolapse and prolapsing hemorrhoids can also be demon-strated in this way. If any discharge is present, cultures can be obtained at this time. Complete examination of the anal canal requires anoscopy.

An acute fissure, a simple crack in the mucosa, will most likely heal after treatment with Sitz baths and stool bulking agents. A chronic fissure has heaped up edges and the fibers of the internal sphincter are often seen at the base of the fissure (Fig. 6.6). If any discharge is present, cultures can be obtained at this time.

Anal condylomata appear as frond-like projections from the perianal skin and anal mucosa. They may occur as a small number of isolated warts or may

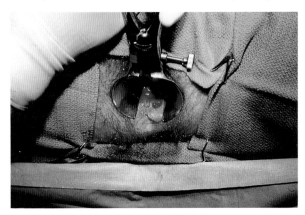

Figure 6.6   Chronic fissure-in-ano.

coalesce and present as a giant mass (Fig. 6.7). Anal condylomata may contain varying degrees of dysplasia up to and including squamous cell carcinoma. The physician may have difficulty distinguishing squamous cell carcinoma from anal condylomata and biopsy is then required to settle the question.

Rectal lymphoma can be confused with perirectal sepsis. A hard, indurated area should arouse suspicion. At operation, a characteristic, fleshy mass is encountered which should be biopsied. The incision should be small and no attempt should be made to excise the lesion. Chemotherapy is the treatment of choice.

Anorectal KS appears as dark, purple lesions which may be located in the perianal skin, in the anal canal or on the rectal mucosa (Fig. 6.8). Biopsy of suspicious lesions will confirm the clinical impression.

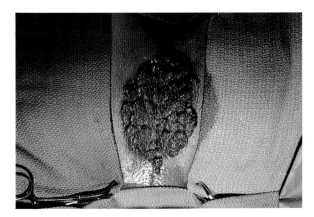

Figure 6.7   Anal condylomata.

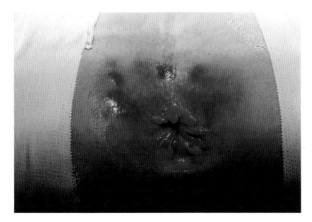

Figure 6.8   Kaposi's sarcoma.

Palpation

There is one basic principle of anorectal examination which needs emphasis: DO NOT HURT THE PATIENT. Wearing two pairs of disposable latex gloves, the lubricated index finger is gently inserted into the anorectum. If the patient's complaint is proctalgia, 5% xylocaine cream can be applied to the anus for a few minutes preceding the digital examination. If the patient experiences severe pain, it is better to stop the examination and discuss the pain; it can then be completed, deferred to another visit or performed in the operating room under anesthesia depending on the circumstances.

Maintain reassuring verbal contact with the patient at all times. Insert the finger gently into the rectum. The tone of the sphincter should be carefully noted; the sphincter tone may have important diagnostic and therapeutic implications. Patients with proctalgia, chronic anal fissure and a very tight sphincter may be candidates for a lateral internal sphincterotomy [33]. The prostate in a man or the cervix in a woman is carefully palpated. The fundus of the uterus can often be felt through the anterior wall of the rectum. The left and right lateral walls of the rectum are then carefully palpated, and finally the hand is rotated 180° so that the posterior wall of the rectum and the hollow of the sacrum is felt. The mucosa is felt for masses, nodules and scarring. Following completion of the digital examination, discard the outer soiled glove and put on a new clean outer glove.

Anoscopy

Although the use of disposable anoscopes for HIV infected patients is appealing, the author has not found a disposable scope which gives good exposure of the anal canal. Our clinic therefore continues to use metal Hirschmann anoscopes which give excellent views of the anal canal.

After gently inserting the anoscope, the obturator is removed allowing exposure of one quadrant of the anal canal. The obturator is carefully reinserted to avoid incorporation of hair or mucosa into the scope. The scope is then rotated 90° and a second quadrant is examined. This process is then repeated until the entire circumference of the anal canal has been inspected. If fulguration of internal anal condylomata is planned, the anal canal should be anesthetized with 5% xylocaine cream prior to anoscopy to allow pain-free fulguration.

Proctosigmoidoscopy

Proctosigmoidoscopy may be performed with either a rigid or flexible fiberoptic sigmoidoscope. The rigid sigmoidoscope may be either reusable or disposable. The disposable variety offers excellent visualization of the colorectal mucosa. Since we perform a large number of proctosig-moidoscopic examinations in patients at high-risk for HIV infection, we use disposable rigid sigmoidoscopes for routine examination in our clinic.

Examination of the unprepared patient can be attempted but is often unrewarding. The patient should be given a Fleet's (R) enema either the night before and on the morning of the examination, or immediately before the examination if the number of patients to be examined and the available facilities permit patient preparation in the clinic.

Digital examination should always precede sigmoidoscopy and anoscopy should usually precede sigmoidoscopy. Failure to do routine anoscopy will result in missed lesions as both the rigid and the flexible fiberoptic sigmoido-scopes give poor views of the anal canal.

After careful insertion of the rigid sigmoidoscope into the rectum, the obturator is removed and the rectal lumen is identified visually. The sigmoidoscope is then gently advanced, always keeping the lumen in view. The sigmoidoscope can almost always be inserted to 15 cm in the prepared patient. Insufflation of a small amount of air may help visualize the rectal lumen. At approximately 15 cm, the rectosigmoid junction is encountered and the lumen can be difficult to find. Slight withdrawal and redirection of the sigmoidoscope combined with air insufflation will often demonstrate the obscure lumen. In some patients, attempts to pass the sigmoidoscope beyond 15 cm results in significant discomfort. Persistent painful attempts to pass the rigid sigmoidoscope are unwise and can result in perforation of the colon or rectum. The sigmoid colon can be evaluated by either a flexible fiberoptic instrument or a barium enema if passage of the rigid sigmoido-scope proves too painful. Patients should not experience significant pain during the examination.

Colorectal biopsy

HIV infected patients with proctitis or colitis may require mucosal biopsy for complete evaluation. Specimens are sent for histopathology and viral cultures. A variety of biopsy forceps are available for trans-sigmoidoscopic biopsy (Fig. 6.9).

Flexible fiberoptic sigmoidoscopy

Flexible fiberoptic sigmoidoscopy should be performed with the patient in the left lateral (Sim's) position. As with rigid sigmoidoscopy, the scope is

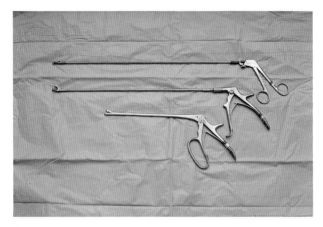

Figure 6.9 Biopsy forceps.

advanced only with a full view of the lumen. In most patients, the colon can be examined to the level of the splenic flexure. Colonic biopsies can be obtained with the flexible biopsy forceps passed through the biopsy channel of the instrument. Following each examination, the flexible fiberoptic sigmoidoscope must be carefully cleaned according to the manufacturer's instructions. We use submersible scopes which are then sterilized in a 2% glutaraldehyde bath for 20 minutes prior to the next examination.

Laboratory examinations

The role of anorectal biopsy and cultures has already been discussed. Patients who have engaged in high-risk sexual behavior should be offered an HIV antibody test as well as a serologic test for syphyllis. Patients who are identified as HIV positive can receive counseling regarding prevention of HIV transmission to others and may be candidates for *Pneumocystis carinii* pneumonia prophylaxis [34] and/or AZT therapy [35].

Summary

HIV infected patients present with anorectal complaints which are either unrelated to their HIV infection, associated with anal intercourse or caused by neoplasia or opportunistic infection directly related to AIDS. A careful history with attention to symptoms and high-risk sexual behavior is important. The physical investigations should include a digital rectal examination, anoscopy and proctoscopy. If a patient experiences significant pain, the examination should be completed in the operating theater under anesthesia. All patients who have engaged in high-risk behavior should be counseled and offered tests for HIV and syphyllis.

References

1. Centers for Disease Control. Public Health Service (PHS) Guidelines for counseling and antibody testing to prevent HIV infection and AIDS. *MMWR* 1987; **36**:509–15.
2. Henry K, Osterholm MT, MacDonald KL. Reduction of HIV transmission by use of condoms. *Am J Public Health* 1988; **78**:1244.
3. Gtzsche PC, Harding M. Condoms to prevent HIV transmission do not imply truly safe sex. *Scand J Infect Dis* 1988; **20**:233–4.
4. Piazza M, Chirianni A, Picciotto L, *et al.* Passionate kissing and microlesions of the oral mucosa: possible role in AIDS transmission. *JAMA* 1989; **261**:244–5.
5. Rogers MF, White CR, Sanders R, *et al.* Lack of transmission of human immunodeficiency virus from infected children to their household contacts. *Pediatrics* 1990; **85**:210–4.
6. Miles AJ, Mellor CH, Gazzard B, *et al.* Surgical management of anorectal disease in HIV-positive homosexuals. *Br J Surg* 1990; **77**:869–71.
7. Carr ND, Mercey D, Slack WW. Non-condylomatous perianal disease in homosexual men. *Br J Surg* 1989; **76**:1064–6.
8. Siegal FP, Lopez C, Hammer GS, *et al.* Severe acquired immunodeficiency in male homosexuals, manifested by chronic perianal ulcerative herpes simplex lesions. *New Engl J Med* 1981; **305**:1439–44.
9. Drew WL, Buhles W, Erlich KS. Herpes virus infections (cytomegalovirus, herpes simplex virus, varicella-zoster virus). How to use ganciclovir (DHPG) and acyclovir. *Infect Dis Clin N Am* 1988; **2**:495–509.
10. Gottesman LG, Miles AJG, Milsom JW, *et al.* The Management of anorectal disease in HIV-positive patients. *Int J Colorect Dis* 1990; **5**:61–72.
11. Law C. Sexually transmitted diseases and enteric infections in the male homosexual population. *Semin Dermatol* 1990; **9**:178–84.
12. Scieux C, Barnes R, Bianchi A, *et al.* Lymphogranuloma venereum: 27 cases in Paris. *J Infect Dis* 1989; **160**:662–8.
13. Stamm WE, Handsfield HH, Rompalo AM, *et al.* The association between genital ulcer disease and acquisition of HIV infection in homosexual men. *JAMA* 1988; **260**:1429–33.
14. Lee MH, Waxman H, Gillooley JF. Primary malignant lymphoma of the anorectum in homosexual men. *Dis Colon Rectum* 1986; **29**:413–16.
15. Lorenz HP, Wilson W, Leigh B, Schecter W. Kaposi's sarcoma of the rectum in AIDS patients. *Arch Surg* (in press).
16. Lorenz HP, Wilson W, Leigh B, *et al.* Squamous cell carcinoma of the anus and HIV infection. *Dis Colon Rectum* (in press).
17. Felt-Bersma RJ, Janssen JJ, Klinkenberg-Knol EC, *et al.* Soiling: anorectal function and results of treatment. *Int J Colon Dis* 1989; **4**:37–40.
18. Heise W, Mostertz P, Arasteh K, *et al.* Gastrointestinal cytomegalovirus manifestations in AIDS. *Gastroenterol* 1989; **27**:725–30.
19. Connolly GM, Shanson D, Hawkins DA, *et al.* Non-cryptosporidial diarrhea in human immunodeficiency virus (HIV) infected patients. *Gut* 1989; **30**:195–200.
20. Connolly GM, Forbes A, Gazzard BG. Investigation of seemingly pathogen negative diarrhea in patients infected with HIV-1. *Gut* 1990; **31**:886–9.
21. Palmer JG, Scholefield JH, Goates PJ, *et al.* Anal cancer and human papillomavirus. *Dis Colon Rectum* 1989; **32**:1016–22.
22. Scholefield JH, Talbor JC, Whatrup C, *et al.* Anal and cervical intraepithelial neoplasia: possible parallel. *Lancet* 1989; **11**:765–9.
23. Navia BA, Jordan BD, Price RW. The AIDS dementia complex. I: Clinical features. *Ann Neurol* 1986; **19**:517–24.

24. Goldstick L, Mandybur TI, Bode R. Spinal cord degeneration in AIDS. *Neurology* 1985; **35**:103–6.
25. Goldschmidt RH, Dong BJ, Johnson MAG, *et al*. Evaluation and treatment of AIDS-associated illnesses: an approach for the primary physician. *J Am Board Fam Pract* 1988; **1**:112–30.
26. Phillips E, Nash P. Culture media. In Lennette EH, Barlows A, Hausler WJ, Shadowy HJ (eds), *Manual of Clinical Microbiology* (4th edn). Washington, DC: American Society for Microbiology, 1985: 1051–92.
27. Centers for Disease Control. Guidelines for prevention of transmission of human immunodeficiency virus and hepatitis B virus to health care and public safety workers. *MMWR* 1989; **38** (no. S-6):3–37.
28. Beck WC. The hole in the surgical glove: a change in attitude. *Bull Am Coll Surg* 1989; **74**:15–16.
29. Gerberding JL, Littell C, Tarkington A, *et al*. Risk of exposure of surgical personnel to patients' blood during surgery at San Francisco General Hospital. *New Engl J Med* 1990; **322**:1788–93.
30. Matta H, Thompson AM, Rainey JB. Does wearing two pairs of gloves protect operating theatre staff from skin contamination? *BMJ* 1988; **297**:597–8.
31. Garden JM, O'Banion MK, Shelnitz LS, *et al*. Papillomavirus in the vapor of carbon dioxide laser-treated verrucae. *JAMA* 1988; **259**:1199–202.
32. Corman ML. Anorectal abscess and fistula. In *Colon and Rectal Surgery*. Philadelphia: Lippincott, 1984: 86–113.
33. Abcarian H. Surgical correction of chronic anal fissure: results of lateral and internal sphincterotomy versus fissurectomy–midline sphincterotomy. *Dis Colon Rectum* 1980; **23**:31–6.
34. Leon GS, Feigal DW, Montgomery AB, *et al*. Aerosolized pentamidine for prophylaxis against pneumocystis carinii pneumonia: the San Francisco community prophylaxis trial. *New Engl J Med* 1990; **323**:769–75.
35. Swart Am, Weller I, Darbyshire JH. Early HIV infection: to treat or not to treat? *BMJ* 1990; **301**:825–6.

MANAGEMENT

7

Proctitis
G Michael Connolly and
David A Hawkins

Introduction

Proctitis may be defined as inflammation of the rectum or anus, but the word is more commonly used to denote rectal mucosal inflammation only. The diagnosis is usually made clinically from the symptoms and the appearance through a proctoscope or sigmoidoscope, with rectal biopsy and appropriate cultures to determine the etiology. Some sexually transmitted infections such as *Neisseria gonorrhoeae* may be present even in the absence of inflammation, and so their presence has been included in the definition of proctitis by some authors [1].

The commonest presentation of acute proctitis is mucopurulent discharge from the anus or, in less severe cases, just mucus streaking of the stool. In addition there may be anorectal bleeding, tenesmus and perianal pain. Locally painful lesions may lead to constipation, as may the sacro-radiculomyelopathy associated with herpetic infections [2]. Abdominal pain and tenderness is suggestive of colitis, and many conditions with more extensive bowel involvement present particularly with diarrhea and are discussed at length below.

In homosexual men most cases of proctitis and proctocolitis are associated with infection with micro-organisms acquired either directly through anal intercourse or alternatively through the fecal–oral route. The former group include *Treponema pallidum*, *N. gonorrhoeae*, *Chlamydia trachomatis* and herpes simplex virus (HSV). The latter group consists of enteric organisms such as *Entamoeba histolytica*, *Shigella*, *Salmonella* and *Campylobacter*. Polymicrobial infection is common [3]; thus an awareness of two or more possible infective agents should be high, as should always be the case when evaluating patients with predominantly sexually transmitted infections. (See Table 7.1.)

Indeed, in the Quinn study published in 1983 about 18% of men with proctitis were infected with two or more organisms or agents. However, it should be noted that the patients studied were attending a sexually transmitted disease clinic (in Seattle) and were therefore a potentially biased sample. Furthermore most were presumably HIV-negative (or at least not particularly immunosuppressed), as the survey was undertaken at the very beginning of the HIV epidemic (1978–81).

Table 7.1   Infections and other conditions found in association with proctitis in HIV-positive men

Bacteria	*Protozoa*
Neisseria gonorrhoeae	*Entamoeba histolytica*
Chlamydia trachomatis	*Giardia lamblia*
(LGV and trachoma biovars)	Cryptosporidia*
Treponema pallidum	*Isospora belli**
Clostridium difficile	Microsporidia*
*Mycobacterium avium intracellulare**	
Enteric bacterial pathogens	*Viruses*
Shigella spp.	Herpes simplex virus
Salmonella spp.	Human papilloma virus
Campylobacter spp.	Cytomegalovirus*
Fungi	*Other conditions*
Candida	Ulcerative proctitis
	Crohn's disease
Helminths	Solitary ulcer syndrome
Enterobius vermicularis	Trauma of anal intercourse
Strongyloides stercoralis	Allergic reactions
	Chemicals and foreign bodies

*Opportunistic infections

Effect of the HIV epidemic

It is now clear that the spread of HIV infection has changed and complicated the clinical picture. This is for two main reasons. First, progressive immunosuppression has led to more diarrheal (enteric) disease and relatively less proctitis. Conditions such as cryptosporidial diarrhea and cytomegalovirus colitis have appeared. In addition, also partly due to immunosuppression, other conditions which may involve the perianal and rectal areas such as Kaposi's sarcoma and non-Hodgkin's lymphoma are occurring and are described elsewhere in this book.

Secondly, changes in sexual behavior in homosexual men, particularly safer sex practices, have been one of the most notable effects of the HIV epidemic. This has led to a remarkable reduction in infections such as rectal gonorrhea in the USA and Europe—although recently there has been a worrying increase in prevalence in younger men [44]. Thus specific infections are still occurring and it is important to undertake specific diagnostic tests (see later).

A survey undertaken by an infectious disease clinic in Baltimore in 1984 and 1985 post-dated the AIDs epidemic and documented some of the above changes. Apart from increased diarrheal disease and less rectal gonorrhea, the survey also noted a decrease in infection due to *Entamoeba histolytica* [4].

Specific types of proctitis

Gonococcal proctitis

Colonization of the rectum by *N. gonorrhoeae* does not necessarily produce signs or symptoms of proctitis. Indeed, several studies have shown that only around 50% of men with uncomplicated rectal gonorrhea are symptomatic. Furthermore, histology of the rectal mucosa may also be negative although there is a mild proctitis with no distinguishing features in some 40% [5].

Examination of stained smears may allow detection of the Gram-negative diplococci, but the test is insensitive at this site (around 60%) and culture of the organism on a selective medium should be performed. Subsequent to culture the isolate may be identified by biochemical or immunological methods. Repeat samples taken a few days later will increase the isolation rate by some 5%. Appropriate swabs should, of course, be taken from other possibly infected sites.

Published reports on treatment for rectal gonorrhea should be treated with caution as the sensitivity profile of the gonococcus is a moving target and varies from year to year and geographically. Current recommendations both nationally (e.g. MMWR) or locally should be followed. The authors' unit currently recommends using ciprofloxacin 500 mg in a single dose by mouth. This dose, which is double that previously recommended, is used as some relative resistance to ciprofloxacin has now been described [6]. Alternative regimens include the penicillins (for sensitive strains), co-trimoxazole and tetracyclines.

It is uncertain whether *Neisseria meningitidis* which is sometimes found in the rectum is pathogenic [7].

Syphilitic (*Treponema pallidum*) proctitis

An anorectal primary chancre may occur within the rectum itself, although they usually present on the perianal skin or within the anal canal. Perianal syphilitic chancres may be painless (like genital lesions elsewhere) and because of their site pass unnoticed. Not infrequently, however, they are painful when they present at the anal margin and thus may be mistaken for trauma or fissures. It is important, therefore, that exudate from these lesions be examined for treponemes by dark-field microscopy or, if this is unavailable, by a monoclonal antibody technique. (In this latter test material is spread on to a glass slide, dried, fixed with acetone and sent to the laboratory.) In addition, blood should be sent for serological tests for syphilis: both a specific test (e.g. TPHA) and a non-specific test (e.g. VDRL) should be performed. These tests may well be negative at the primary stage and need to be repeated, although HIV-positive patients may not develop the characteristic fourfold or more rise in antibody titer owing to a defective response to neoantigens [8]. Primary syphilis of the rectum may present with symptoms of proctitis and have the appearance of hypertrophic lesions sometimes with central ulceration. In addition, secondary syphilis has also been described as causing a diffuse distal proctitis. Biopsy is said to be contraindicated because of the risk of severe hemorrhage, but when it is performed the histology has been recorded as showing intense lympho-plasmacytic infiltration in the lamina propria, the presence of granulomata and giant cell formation with crypt distortion but no abscesses [9].

Standard therapy for syphilis includes procaine penicillin 600 000 units daily for 10 days IM, or benzathine penicillin 2.4 mega-units IM repeated after one week. However, there have been several reports of reactivation of syphilis after seemingly adequate therapy in HIV-positive patients [10]. It is probably wise in this group to consider using longer courses of treatment, such as daily procaine penicillin for 21 days, in the hope of preventing relapse or the development of more serious disease such as neurologic syphilis. Patients allergic to penicillin can be treated with tetracyclines (300 mg of doxycyline daily in divided doses for 21 days).

Non-syphilitic spirochetal organisms are commonly found in homosexual men causing a condition called intestinal spirochetosis [9]. There is no evidence to date that these organisms are pathogenic in either HIV-positive or HIV-negative patients.

Chlamydia trachomatis proctitis

Chlamydiae are obligate intracellular parasites which are very widespread in nature. There are two biovars, trachoma and lymphogranuloma vene-reum (LGV). It is thought that most hyperendemic trachoma is caused by the A, B, and C serovars, whereas the D to K serovars are responsible for the numerous manifestations of chlamydiae such as inclusion conjunctivitis and the various genital infections. The trachoma biovar can also infect the rectum, but it is not clear whether it is a cause of proctitis as, in a number of studies [11], well over half the patients had no symptoms or signs of proctitis. LGV serovars appear to be relatively uncommon in temperate climes but may cause severe proctitis, particularly when directly inoculated into the rectum as in homosexual contact. In one study by Schacter looking at isolates of chlamydiae from the rectum of patients with severe proctitis, 20 out of 27 strains were LGV serovars [12].

The incubation period for LGV is thought to be between a few days and a few weeks and we have seen it develop 10 days after rectal gonorrhea had been successfully treated (with spectinomycin). Early symptoms of rectal LGV are purulent discharge and bleeding with the possible later develop-ment of gross inguinal lymphadenopathy so characteristic of the disease. Sigmoidoscopy reveals a distal proctitis maybe extending beyond 15 cm, and ulcerative or hypertrophic forms have been described. Biopsy may reveal an 'infective' proctitis with increased plasma cells and poly-morphonuclear leukocytes with crypt abscesses, or there may be granulomas and giant cells present. The histology may be confused with either Crohn's disease or even ulcerative colitis. When a proctitis is found with colonization with non-LGV chlamydial strains it is usually mild. It is likely that histology may be atypical in HIV disease as granuloma formation may be impaired.

Diagnosis is preferably made by culture either from a rectal swab or biopsy specimen. This requires the availability of an appropriate transport medium and transfer to an experienced laboratory. Alternatively non-cultural tests can be performed using monoclonals in an ELISA test or linked to fluorescein for direct immunofluorescent tests [13]. These, however, have not been well validated as diagnostic tests from the rectum. With respect to LGV proctitis, a typical clinical picture associated with a strongly positive complement fixation test titer greater than 1/16 strongly supports the diagnosis. Again, however, it must be remembered that serologic responses may be impaired in HIV disease.

As with all chlamydial infections, tetracyclines are the drugs of choice and should be given for at least 2–3 weeks. Appropriate regimens are oxytetracycline 500 mg four times a day orally, or doxycycline 100 mg twice a day. Other drugs that have been advocated are rifampicin, which is extremely active against the chlamydiae but probably should be reserved for tuberculous infections, sulphonamides, which are less active *in vitro*, and erythromycin. More recently some of the quinolones such as ofloxacin have been shown to have good activity [14]. Finally, anal stricture is usually a late complication of LGV infection and may require surgical treatment.

Anorectal warts

These are discussed at length elsewhere. At times they may not be visible with the naked eye, but they nevertheless cause proctitis and thus need to be considered in the differential diagnosis.

Herpetic proctitis

Genital herpes reached epidemic proportions in the USA and latterly in the UK prior to the HIV epidemic. Subsequently it became apparent that many homosexual men, as they became more immunosuppressed, were getting frequent attacks of perianal herpes, suggesting that this infection was indeed very common in this group. In addition to the classical presentation with painful vesicles perianally, which later ulcerate, there may also be a proctitis with edema and discrete focal ulceration but no vesicle formation. This usually causes symptoms such as rectal bleeding, discharge and rectal pain, but may be totally asymptomatic.

Helminthic infections

Enterobius vermicularis, or pinworm, is a fairly common infestation in homosexual men and may be acquired by anilingus. Pruritis ani due to the deposition of ova is the commonest symptom although adult female worms may be seen incidentally in the stools or by proctoscopy. The diagnosis is made by demonstrating the ova collected on transparent adhesive tape from the anal area. Treatment regimens with mebendazole or piperazine are effective.

Strongyloides stercoralis can produce an ulcerative colitis and may possibly reactivate in an immunocompromised patient.

Traumatic and iatrogenic proctitis

A vast array of objects may be inserted into the rectum for sexual gratification and may cause variable degrees of trauma, including proctitis. Furthermore, penoreceptive intercourse alone may cause clinical proctitis on the anterior wall of the rectum [1]. In the context of the AIDS era there are anecdotal reports that various lubricants containing spermacides such as nonoxynol-9, which are toxic to HIV, may on occasion cause rectal inflammation.

Diarrheal diseases

Diarrhea is a major manifestation of HIV disease and virtually all patients will develop diarrhea at some stage in the course of their illness [15]. In the early years of the epidemic a specific cause for diarrhea was found in only about one-third of patients, but as our knowledge has progressed and laboratory experience developed it is now possible to identify a potential pathogen in 70% of patients. Proctitis and rectal pathology may not always be a major feature, of course, but sigmoidoscopy and rectal biopsy are often abnormal and are of considerable value in diagnosis. Conversely it is unusual to make additional diagnoses with double-contrast barium enemas or at colonoscopy [16].

Importance of the stage of HIV disease

Assessing the severity and the stage of HIV disease may be helpful in diagnosis. In particular, a consistently low CD4 positive lymphocyte (T-helper cell) count is useful as infections such as persistent cryptosporidial diarrhea, disseminated *Mycobacterium avium intracellulare* (MAI) infection and disseminated CMV are rarely found in patients with counts above 50–100/ml^3.

Severe weight loss may also be indicative of the above three pathogens, and very-high-volume diarrhea suggests cryptosporidial infection [17].

Routine hematology may also be helpful. Development of anemia which cannot be attributed to a side-effect of myelosuppressive drug therapy may be due to disseminated MAI infection [18].

Cryptosporidia

Cryptosporidium parvum is a parasitic protozoa which was first described as causing disease in man in 1976 [19]. Subsequently it has proved to be a common cause of acute infective gastroenteritis. In immunocompetent individuals it causes a diarrheal disease with crampy abdominal pains which is self-limiting and lasts for less than two weeks. However, in immunocompromised patients, including those with AIDS, it may produce severe protracted diarrhea (up to 15 liters per day) with weight loss and inanition, and it may be life-threatening [20,21]. Subsequently, with increasing recognition and improved diagnostic tests, most patients have been found to have between one and three liters of stool per day with weight loss of 5–10 kg at the time of diagnosis [22]. The diarrhea is characteristically watery and abdominal pain is not a major feature except perhaps terminally.

Diagnosis is made by examining stool specimens using a modified acid-fast stain. Numerous stool samples and the use of a concentration method may be required if there are small numbers of oocysts. Sigmoidoscopy may reveal a non-specific proctitis, and histology of rectal biopsy can lead to identification of the organisms (Fig. 7.1).

As yet no drug has been found to be effective against cryptosporidia, although anecdotal reports of improvement have been reported with macrolide antibiotics such as spiramycin and erythromycin. Zidovudine, perhaps by leading to some improvement in the immune status of patients, sometimes produces a marked improvement in diarrhea with loss of oocysts from the stool [22]. Unfortunately many patients subsequently relapse while still on treatment. This, however, may be after a period of some months of good-quality life.

Isospora

Isospora belli is another protozoa parasite primarily affecting the small intestine which has a life-cycle and clinical effect similar to cryptosporidia [23]. Although less common than the latter in most populations, it is important to recognize as it appears to respond well to trimethoprim plus sulphamethoxazole. Diagnosis is by modified Ziehl–Neelsen strains of the stool, revealing acid-fast oocysts much larger at 20–$30\,\mu$m (cf. 2–$5\,\mu$m) than those of cryptosporidia.

Microsporidia

Microsporidia are small protozoan parasites that are increasingly being found in AIDS patients with otherwise unexplained diarrhea. Diagnosis used to require electron microscopy of small bowel biopsies. However, with an experienced histopathologist light microscopy of low duodenal biopsies are equally sensitive and specific [45]. The microorganisms have recently been detected in stool [24] but have not been seen on rectal biopsy.

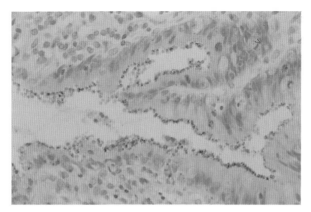

Figure 7.1 Rectal biopsy (glycogen stain) showing surface cryptosporidia.

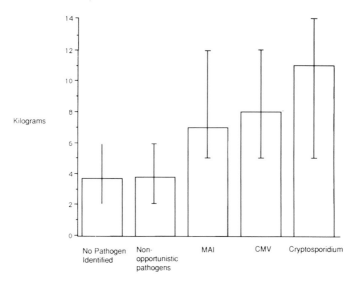

Figure 7.2 Average weight loss in various groups at presentation.

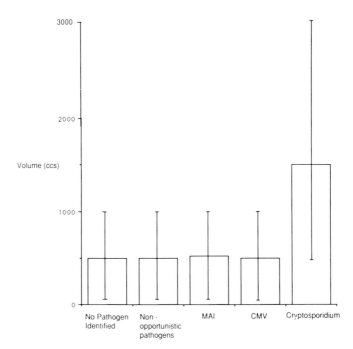

Figure 7.3 Average daily stool volumes in various groups at presentation.

Cytomegalovirus

Cytomegalovirus (CMV), like all herpes viruses, can cause primary, latent, or chronic persistent infections. CMV is now recognized as a major cause of gastrointestinal symptoms in HIV-positive patients including oesophagitis, gastritis, enteritis and colitis [25–27]. Perianal and perioral disease also occurs [28]. The most common presenting manifestations of CMV colitis are diarrhea and abdominal pain occurring in 100% and 82% of patients respectively [30]. Up to twenty liquid motions per day can occur with intermittent or continuous abdominal pain and symptoms which mimic diverticulitis, intra-abdominal abscess or ischemia.

Patients may also present as an acute surgical emergency with severe bleeding per rectum, toxic dilatation and possibly perforation [30]. Weight loss can be severe (Fig. 7.2) and the majority of patients are anemic and some have rebound tenderness. CMV colitis almost always presents as a pan colitis; (thus examination of the rectum will reveal non-specific proctitis similar to inflammatory bowel disease (Fig. 7.4)), although occasionally as isolated ulceration. Examination of histological specimens including those from rectal biopsy may reveal characteristic inclusion bodies surrounded by acute and chronic inflammatory cells. More recently immunoperoxidase staining has been used (Fig. 7.5) and it appears that this may be a useful adjunct in patients who have lower numbers of CMV inclusions [32]. CMV colitis may mimic inflammatory bowel disease (IBD), or pre-existing bowel disease may suddenly deteriorate when superinfection with CMV occurs in the presence of HIV disease [32]. Conversely IBD may improve after HIV infection [33].

There are now two recognized drugs for the treatment of CMV disease. Foscarnet has been licensed in some countries and is at present undergoing

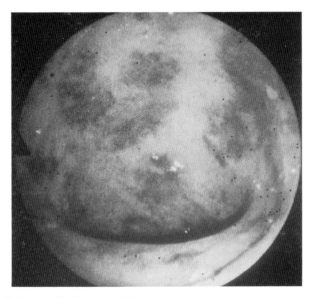

Figure 7.4 Cytomegalovirus proctitis.

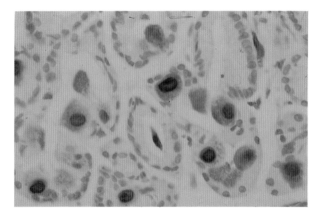

Figure 7.5   Immunoflourescent stain showing cytomegalovirus in rectal biopsy.

extensive trials in the USA, whereas ganciclovir (DHPG) is a drug long established to be of value in the treatment of CMV disease of the retina and gastrointestinal tract [30]. There are major drawbacks to the use of both drugs in that they both have to be administered intravenously, usually via a central line. Foscarnet may cause irreversible renal failure which may be reduced by prehydration [34]. In addition, complex changes in calcium homeostasis may occur. In about 10% of patients the serum calcium rises above the normal, and in a further 10% it falls below the normal range. Recent studies indicate that the CMV infection of the eye has been successfully treated by foscarnet, and this is also true of CMV infection of the gut despite an early negative report [35,36,43]. A major side-effect of ganciclovir is bone marrow suppression which may be a particular problem in patients taking AZT. A reduction in dosage and interruption of treatment are commony required when a neutrophil count falls below 500×10^9 per liter.

Both ganciclovir and foscarnet are virostatic agents and relapse of clinical symptoms appears common where therapy is interrupted. Thus life-long treatment may be required. Interpretation of the effectiveness of therapy in CMV colitis is complicated by the fact that these patients often have dual (or triple) pathology, most often with cryptosporidiosis.

Mycobacterium avium intracellulare

MAI may cause fever and anemia associated with an abnormal bone marrow. It usually causes a disseminated infection and it is interesting to note that at autopsy it is found somewhere within the body in virtually 100% of AIDS patients. Its significance therefore is uncertain.

Despite this MAI is found in a small percentage of AIDS patients with diarrhea and, although appearances in the rectal mucosa are non-specific, the diagnosis may be made on occasion by rectal biopsy or by finding the organism in the stool [37].

Although MAI appears to be sensitive *in vitro* to a range of antituberculous drugs, the response *in vivo* has been disappointing with little effect on stool volumes in diarrheal disease [38].

Salmonella

Salmonellosis due to *Salmonella typhimurium*, an intracellular organism, appears to be a quite common infection in AIDS patients. The defect in cellular immune response may lead to a severe systemic infection with bacteremia. Presentation as an abdominal emergency with toxic dilatation of the colon has been described. Diagnosis is by stool and blood cultures, and appearances at sigmoidoscopy and on rectal biopsy are non-specific. Because of the severe disease antibiotic treatment is warranted with drugs such as ciprofloxacin depending on local sensitivity testing. Furthermore recurrence of disease is commonplace on discontinuation of therapy, so long-term suppressive therapy should be considered [39].

Shigella

Prior to the AIDS epidemic, shigellosis had been noted to be venereally transmitted and quite common in homosexual men. *Shigella sonnei* usually causes a mild colonic inflammation; *S. flexneri* strains more likely involve the rectum or sigmoid colon [1]. A pseudomembranous colitis has been described [38]. In AIDS patients, as with Salmonella infection a systemic disease with bacteremia may occur along with a tendency to relapse [40]. Early and prolonged therapy with appropriate antibiotics is therefore required.

Campylobacter

Campylobacter species are curved Gram-negative motile bacilli which are often seen in the stools of homosexual men with proctitis, including those with HIV infection. Apart from *C. jejuni* their pathogenicity is uncertain. Recent reports have described Campylobacter-like organisms in HIV-positive men less frequently than previously, but they may be associated with bacteremia [4].

Giardia

Giardia infection is common in homosexual men and may produce a discrete ulceration in the colon of AIDS patients. Attempts at fecal isolation may be negative and diagnosis only achieved by examination of a duodenal aspirate or jejunal biopsy. In view of this, treatment with metronidazole or tinidazole at an early stage of diarrheal disease in HIV-positive patients is recommended.

Amebae

Various species of amebae may inhabit the intestine although most are almost invariably non-pathogenic (*Entamoeba hartmanni, Entamoeba coli*,

Dientamoeba fragilis, Iodamoeba buetschlii and *Endolimax nana*). *Entamoeba histolytica* may, of course, produce symptomatic amebiasis with large bowel or rectal inflammation which may be complicated by liver abscess. However, in most homosexual men *E. histolytica* appears to act as a commensal, the organisms lacking the ability to invade the mucosa. There has been an extended debate as to whether these so called 'non-pathogenic' zymodenes of *E. histolytica* may be associated with proctitis. Most authors have found no association with symptoms, although McMillan and others found histologic evidence of proctitis more often in those infected with *E. histolytica* than those uninfected [41,42]. There is no evidence to date that the immuno-compromised state of HIV infection allows these 'non-pathogenic' zymodenes to become pathogenic. Furthermore, changing sexual practices may have led to a decreased prevalence of these organisms[4].

Summary

There are clearly a large number of possible causes of proctitis in HIV-positive men. Specific etiologies including predominantly sexually transmitted agents need to be considered as safe sex cannot be assumed. However, presentations may be atypical because of altered immune responses. Many other conditions, particularly the protean causes of diarrhea in this group, may have a proctitic component although the appearances by naked eye and histologically may well be non-specific. Diagnosis will be aided by considering the overall clinical picture, including the degree of immunosuppression and evidence of disease at other sites.

References

1. Goldmeier D. Proctitis. In Taylor-Robinson D (ed), *Clinical Problems in Sexually Transmitted Diseases*. Amsterdam: Martinus Nijhoff, 1985: 15–35.
2. Samarasinghe PL, Oates JK, MacLennon IBP. Herpetic proctitis and sacral radiculomyelopathy: a hazard for homosexual men. *Br Med J* 1979; **2**:365.
3. Quinn TC, Stamm WE, Goodell SE, *et al.* The polymicrobial origin of intestinal infections in homosexual men. *New Engl J. Med* 1983; **309**:576.
4. Laughon Barbara E, Druckman DA, Vernon A, *et al.* Prevalence of enteric pathogens in homosexual men with and without acquired immunodeficiency syndrome. *Gastroenterology* 1988; **94**:984–93.
5. McMillan A, McNeillage G, Gilmour H, Lee FD. Histology of rectal gonorrhoea in men, with a note on anorectal infection with *Neisseria meningitidis. J Clin Path* 1983; **36**:511–14.
6. Grandsden WR, Warren CA, Phillips I, Hodges M, Barlow D. Decreased susceptibility of *Neisseria gonorrhoeae* to ciprofloxacin. *Lancet* 1990; **335** (8680): 51.
7. Janda WM, Bohnhoff M, Morello JA, Lerner SA. Prevalence and site pathogen studies of *Neisseria meningitidis* and *Neisseria gonorrhoeae* in homosexual men. *JAMA* 1980; **244**:2060–64.
8. Hicks CB, Benson PM, Lupton GP, Tramont EC, Spence MR, Abrutyn E. Seronegative secondary syphilis in a patient infected with the human immunodeficiency virus (HIV) with Kaposi's sarcoma: a diagnostic dilemma. *Ann Int Med* 1987; **107** (4): 492–4.

9. McMillan A, Lee FD. Sigmoidoscopic and microscopic appearance of the rectal mucosa in homosexual men. *Gut* 1981; **22**: 1035–41.
10. Berry CD, Hooton JM, Collier AC, Lukehart SA. Neurological relapse after benzathine penicillin therapy for secondary syphilis in a patient with HIV infection. *New Engl J Med* 1987; **316**: 1587–9.
11. Munday PE, Dawson SG Johnson AP, *et al*. A microbiological study of non-gonococcal proctitis in passive male homosexuals. *Postgrad Med J*. 1981; **57**: 705–11.
12. Schachter T, Osoba AO. Lymphogranuloma venereum. In: Chlamydial disease *Br Med Bull* 1983; **39** (2): 151–4.
13. Rompalo AM, Suchland RJ, Price CB, Stamm WE. Rapid diagnosis of *Chlamydia trachomatis* rectal infection by direct immunofluorescence staining. *J Infect Dis* 1987; **155**:1075.
14. Batteiger BE, Jones RB, White A. Efficacy and safety of ofloxacin in the treatment of nongonococcal sexually transmitted disease. *Am J Med* 1989; **87** (6C): 75S–77S.
15. Connolly GM, Shanson D, Hawkins DA, *et al*. Non-cryptosporidial diarrhoea in human immunodeficiency virus (HIV) infected patients. *Gut* 1989; **30**:195–200.
16. Connolly GM, Forbes A, Gleeson JA, Gazzard BG. The value of barium enema and colonoscopy in patients infected with HIV. *AIDS* 1990; **4**:687–9.
17. Connolly GM, Dryden MS, Shanson DC, Gazzard BG. Cryptosporidial diarrhoea in AIDS and its treatment. *Gut* 29:593–7.
18. Gardner TD, Flanagan P, Dryden MI, *et al*. Disseminated mycobacterium avium-intercellulare infection and red cells hypoplasia in patients with the acquired immune deficiency syndrome. *J Infect* 1988; **16**:135–40.
19. Nime FA, Burch JD, Page DL, *et al*. Acute enterocolitis in a human being infected with the protozoan *Cryptosporidium*. *Gastroenterology* 1976; **70**: 592–8.
20. Soave R, Johnson WD. *Cryptosporidium* and *Isospora belli* infections. *J. Infect Dis* 1988; **157**:225–9.
21. Navin TR, Hardy AM. Crytosporidiosis in patients with AIDS. *J. Inf. Dis* 1987; **155**:150.
22. Connolly GM. Clinical aspects of cryptosporidiosis. *Ballière's Clinical Gastroenterology* 4 No 2, June 1990.
23. Shein R, Gell A. *Isospora belli* in a patient with acquired immune deficiency syndrome. *J Clin Gastroent* 1984; **6**: 525.
24. Van Goo LT, Hollister WS, Schattenkerh JE, *et al*. Diagnosis of *Enterocytozoon bieneusi* microsporidiosis in AIDS patients by recovery of spores from faeces. Lancet 1990; **336**: 697–8.
25. Knapp AB, Horst DA, Elypolos G, *et al*. Widespread cytomegalovirus gastro-enterocolitis in a patient with acquired immune deficiency syndrome. *Gastroenterology* 1983; **85**: 1399–402.
26. Freedman PG, Werner BC, Balthazar ES. Cytomegalovirus oesphagogastritis in a patient with acquired immunodeficiency syndrome. *Am J Gastroenterol* 1985; **80**: 434–7.
27. Meiselman MS, Cello JS, Margaretten W. Cytomegalovirus colitis: report of the clinical, endoscopic and pathological findings on two patients with acquired immunodeficiency syndrome. *Gastroenterology* 1985; **88**: 171–5.
28. Connolly GM. Cytomegalovirus disease in AIDS. *Baillière's Clinical Gastroenterology* 4, No. 2, June 1990.
29. Connolly GM. Cytomegalovirus infection of the gastrointestinal tracts of patients with HIV-1 or AIDS. *J Clin Pathol* 1989; **42**:1055–64.
30. Jacobson MA, Mills J. Serious cytomegalovirus disease in the acquired immunodeficiency syndrome (AIDS): clinical findings, diagnosis and treatment. *Ann Int Med* 1988; **108**:585–94.
31. Francis ND, Bolyston AWB, Roberts AHG, *et al*. Cytomegalovirus infection of

the gastrointestinal tracts of patients infected with HIV-1 or AIDS. *J Clin Pathol* **42**:1055–64.

32. Liebowitz D, McShane D. Non-specific chronic inflammatory bowel disease and AIDS. *J. Clin Gasterenterol* 1986; **8** (1):66– 8.

33. James SP. Remission of Chrohn's disease after human immunodeficiency virus infection. *Gastroenterology* 1988; **95**: 1667–9.

34. Deray G, Franck M, Katlama C, *et al*. Foscarnet nephrotoxicity: mechanism, incidence and preventions. *Am J Nephrol* 1989; **9**:316–21.

35. Moyle G, Mathalone B, Gazzard B. An open randomised comparative study of foscarnet and Ganciclovir in the treatment of CMV retinitis. Abstract FB95, VIth Conference on AIDS, 1990.

36. Weber JN, Thom S, Barrison T. Cytomegalovirus colitis and oesophageal ulceration in the context of AIDS: clinical manifestations and preliminary report of treatment with foscarnet (phosphonoformate). *Gut* 1987; **28**:482–7.

37. Horsburg CR, Mason VG, Farhi DC. Disseminated infection with mycobacterium avium intercellulare: a report of 13 cases and a review of the literature. *Medicine* 1985; **64**:36–48.

38. Gazzard, HIV disease and the gastroenterologist. *Gut* 1988; **29**:1497–505.

39. Jacobs JL, Gold JWM, Murray MW, *et al*. Salmonella infection in patients with the acquired immunodeficiency syndrome. *Ann Intern Med* 1985; **102**:86.

40. Baskin DH, Lax JD, Barenberg D. Shigella bacteremia in patients with the acquired immune deficiency syndrome. *Am J Gastroenterol* 1987; **82**:338.

41. Goldmeier D, Sargeant PG, Price AJ, *et al*. Is *Entamoeba histolytica* in homosexual men a pathogen? *Lancet* 1986; 641–4.

42. McMillan A, Gilmour HM, McNeillage G. Amoebiasis in homosexual men. *Gut* 1984; **25**: 356–60.

43. Nelson M, Connolly GM, Hawkins DA, Gazzard BG.

44. Singaralram AE, Boag F, Barton SE, Hawkins DA, Laurence AG. Preventing the spread of HIV infection. *Brit. Med. J.* (1991); **302**:469.

45. Peacock CS, Blanchard C, Ellis DS, Tovey DG, Gazzard BG. The histological diagnosis of intestinal microsponda in AIDS. *J. Clin, Palv.* (1991); (in press).

8

Anal and rectal ulceration
Maria Elena Soler and Lester Gottesman

Introduction

Recent studies showing the strong association between HIV seropositivity and ulcerative diseases place futher importance on the timely diagnosis and appropriate treatment of anal ulcers [1–3]. Anal fissures commonly affect both healthy and immunocompromised patients. Normally, these tears in the anal canal are initiated by the passage of hard stools. The most common site for a benign fissure is the anteroposterior vertical axis of the anus, and it has been suggested that this is due to the relationship of the surrounding anal sphincters to the posterior angulation of the rectum [4]. Anal sphincter manometry has shown that the maximum resting pressure is significantly higher in patients with anal fissures, suggesting hypertonicity of the internal sphincter to be a major contributing factor [5,6]. Consequently, internal sphincterotomy, which permanently reduces anal sphincter pressure, allows subsequent healing of the fissure [7–10].

Immunocompromised patients pose a diagnostic and therapeutic problem, since they are susceptible to a wider range of diseases that may present as anal ulcerations. Homosexual men may present with traumatic fissures related to their sexual practices [11]. Many HIV-positive patients suffer from chronic diarrhea, which has been recognized as another etiologic factor in the development of benign fissures. These fissures act as other benign fissures; that is, they are in the midline, are associated with sentinal tags and a hypertonic sphincter. Treating these patients surgically presents a difficult problem since sphincterotomy may lead to incontinence in patients unable to have formed bowel movements. In addition to benign fissures, HIV-positive patients are often afflicted with pathologic ulcerative processes that extend above the dentate line, invade deep into the anal sphincters, and are not located in the anteroposterior axis. In contrast to benign fissures, these chronic ulcerations are not typically associated with increased pressure in the anal canal. With the homosexual AIDS patient, the clinician must not only recognize traumatic and idiopathic fissures but must also be aware of the myriad of infectious and neoplastic conditions that masquarade as anal ulcers. Establishing the etiology of anal fissures and ulcers in immunocompromised patients is a difficult and tedious task. In this chapter, we discuss the diagnosis and treatment of idiopathic, traumatic and infectious ulcers in immunocompromised patients. The neoplastic disorders associated with anal ulcers will be mentioned here but are covered in more detail in Chapter 11.

A number of infectious etiologies of anal ulcerations may be seen in immunocompetent homosexual men, HIV-positive and AIDS patients. The infectious disorders can be divided into bacterial, viral, fungal, and parasitic diseases.

Bacterial infections

Tuberculosis

Tuberculosis is an infectious, communicable, bacterial disease, caused by *Mycobacterium tuberculosis*. In 1986, the number of reported cases of tuberculosis in the USA increased for the first time in 30 years, probably as a result of the HIVepidemic [12]. The association of AIDS with tuberculosis is now clearly recognized, and seems to be related to certain risk groups. AIDS patients who were black, of foreign origin, or had a history of intravenous drug abuse, were more likely to have tuberculosis [13]. In Florida, tuberculosis was diagnosed before AIDS in over 70% of cases. A number of studies have confirmed that AIDS patients are more likely to have extrapulmonary manifestations of the disease. Tuberculosis of the anal canal may manifest itself as ulcers or fissures.

Tuberculosis is primarily transmitted via the respiratory system, through inhalation of aerosolized droplets of the bacillus. Infection via the gastrointestinal tract or by penetration of intact skin or mucosa has been described, and may be an important mode of transmission in homosexual men [14]. The bacilli spread through the lymphatic channels to the regional lymph nodes and through the blood stream to more distant sites. In the immunocompetent host, acquired immunity develops over several weeks and limits the multiplication and spread of the bacillus. At this point the patient develops a positive PPD (purified protein derivative), a cutaneous manifestation of the delayed hypersensitivity reaction to the tuberculin bacillus. With the persistence of viable bacilli in foci throughout the body, the host maintains a degree of protection against future tuberculosis infections. However, if the individual becomes immunosuppressed, the disease may be reactivated many years after the initial infection. It seems most likely that this is the mechanism by which HIV infected patients develop tuberculosis [15].

Establishing the diagnosis in immunocompromised patients is not always straightforward and may require the use of several modalities before one gets a positive result. A tuberculin skin test may suggest the presence of infection. However, one may get a false-positive test from cross-reactivity with other non-tuberculous mycobacteria. On the other hand, patients who are immunosuppressed may not be able to mount a delayed hypersensitivity response. Only 10–40% of HIV infected patients will have a positive tuberculin skin test at the time of the diagnosis of tuberculosis [16,17]. The tuberculin test of choice is the intradermal injection of 5 TU of tuberculin PPD stabilized with polysorbate 80. In the USA, 0.1 ml of the commercially available preparations Aplisol or Tubersol contain the adequate mixture [14].

Grossly, these lesions are superficial circumferential ulcers with their long axis perpendicular to the lumen, leading to strictures and stenosis as they heal. Histologically, granuloma formation is seen, sometimes with caseation. In addition, microscopic examination for acid-fast bacilli, using a Ziehl–Neelsen stain, should be performed on all specimens. The 'gold standard' for diagnosis is culture of the organism. Biopsy specimens of anal ulcers should be sent for culture, as well as pathology. More recently, labeled-DNA probes specific for ribosomal RNA have been used to detect *M. tuberculosis* [18].

In general, patients coinfected with tuberculosis and HIV respond well to standard antituberculosis drugs, although they may need a longer course of therapy. The recommended regimen is isoniazid (10–15 mg/kg/day up to 300 mg/day), rifampin (10–15 mg/kg/day up to 600 mg/day), and either pyrazinamide (20–30 mg/kg/day) or ethambutol (25 mg/kg/day). The last two drugs are only given during the first two months of treatment. Treatment should be continued for at least 6 months after documented culture conversion, but for a minimum of 9 months altogether. If either isoniazid or rifampicin is not used, therapy should be continued for 12 months after culture conversion, but for a minimum of 18 months in total.

Syphilis

Syphilis is a sexually transmitted disease caused by the spirochete *Treponema pallidum*. During the mid-1970s and early 1980s, syphilis became almost pandemic in the male homosexual population. However, with the advent of the AIDS epidemic and the concomitant change in the sexual practices of homosexual men, there has been a decrease in the incidence of syphilis in this group [19,20]. Still, several studies have shown that patients with reactive syphilis serology have a higher risk of having antibodies to HIV. Therefore, every patient with positive syphilis serology should be tested for HIV antibodies and vice versa. There is also growing evidence that syphilis may facilitate the acquisition and activation of HIV. Some studies suggest that all genital ulcers facilitate the transmission of HIV, by disruption of the cutaneous barrier to HIV. Others believe that the immunologic response to the spirochete infection leads to the antigenic stimulation of latently HIV-infected cells, resulting in activation and liberation of HIV [21,22].

Approximately three weeks after infection, a chancre forms at the site where inoculation took place. The classic primary chancre is typically a single, painless papule which quickly erodes to form an ulcer with a smooth base and firm, raised borders (Fig. 8.1). These ulcers are usually painless but may cause rectal pain, tenesmus, difficulty with defecation, and rectal discharge. Although the condition can be easily confused with a benign fissure, an aberrant location, such as the lateral anal margin, should raise suspicion. The primary lesion is associated with the presence of firm, non-suppurative, painless inguinal lymphadenopathy.

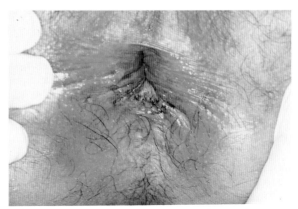

Figure 8.1   Syphilitic ulcer in HIV-positive patient (note adjacent condylomta).

Dark-field examination is the quickest and most direct way to make the diagnosis of syphilis. The serous transudate from a moist lesion is the most productive since these lesions have the greatest number of treponemes. The surface of the suspected lesion should be cleansed with saline and gently abraded with a dry gauze so as not to produce gross bleeding. The serous exudate can then be squeezed on to a glass slide, covered with a coverslip, and examined with dark-field or phase-contrast microscopy. *T. pallidum* will have a corkscrew appearance and move in a spiraling motion with a characteristic undulation about its midpoint. Only after three negative examinations can the lesion be considered non-syphilitic. A topical antiseptic will kill the organism, necessitating the use of direct or indirect immunoflourescent or immunoperoxidase staining [23]. Biopsy of the ulcer can also be helpful, demonstrating a mononuclear infiltrate in the floor and the margin of the ulcer. Spirochetes can be seen with a Warthin–Starry stain [24]. Specific immunoflourescent or immunoperoxidase staining of non-frozen pathologic specimens has also been described [25,26].

Serologic testing has been the cornerstone for the diagnosis and follow-up of patients with syphilis. It appears that most HIV-positive patients have normal serologic responses to *T. pallidum*. Therefore, it remains the diagnostic tool of choice. Two different types of antibodies are measured: the non-specific non-treponemal reaginic antibody and the specific antitreponemal antibody. A variety of non-treponemal tests are available. They are inexpensive, rapid, convenient for screening large numbers of patients, and helpful in monitoring disease activity. Syphilis reaginic antibodies are IgG and IgM immunoglobulins directed against a lipoidal antigen that is the result of the interaction of the host tissue with *T. pallidum*. The standard non-treponemal test is the Venereal Disease Research Laboratory (VDRL) slide test, which tests heated serum for its ability to flocculate a suspension of cardiolipin–cholesterol–lecithin antigen. It is useful in monitoring a patient's response to treatment. A persistent positive VDRL, after adequate treatment, may indicate a persistent active infection or reinfection, especially if the titer is greater than 1:4. It may also, however, be a false reaction. There are two modifications of the VDRL available for routine screening: the rapid plasma reagin card test (RPR) and the automated reagin test (ART). The quantitative RPR should become non-reactive in primary syphilis one year after successful treatment, two years after secondary syphilis and five years after treatment for late syphilis. If the RPR remains elevated after the appropriate interval of time has elapsed, it suggests a persistent infection, reinfection or a false-positive test. Specific antitreponemal antibody tests are used to confirm the diagnosis, since it establishes the high likelihood of a treponemal infection at the present time or in the past. Once positive it remains positive for life. The most common specific antitreponemal antibody test done today is the flourescent treponemal antibody absorption test (FTA-bas). It is a standard indirect immunoflourescent antibody test that uses *T. pallidum* harvested from rabbit testes as the antigen. As with most other immunoflourescent tests it is standardized at one dilution, is difficult to quantitate, and varies from one laboratory to the next. Therefore, the interpretation is quite subjective and requires great attention to detail The *T. pallidum* hemagglutination assay (TPHA-TP) also measures specific treponemal antibodies. Although less sensitive in early disease, it is easier to perform and is as sensitive as the FTA-abs. For all practical purposes they are interchangable. Negative serology does not exclude the diagnosis, since serologic tests do not become positive until the primary chancre has been present for several weeks. In addition, immunocompromised patients may have a prolonged interval between infection and seroconversion [14]. However, in the anal lesions of secondary syphilis serologic tests are virtually always positive.

Because syphilis has a wide range of clinical manifestations, it is difficult to assess the frequency of unusual clinical and laboratory manifestations of syphilis in patients co-infected with HIV. Although most HIV infected patients seem to have a normal serologic response to *T. pallidum* infection, there have been cases of biopsy-proven secondary syphilis infection with negative treponemal and non-treponemal tests [27,28]. In March 1988, the CDC published some guidelines for the diagnosis and treatment of syphilis in HIV-infected patients. They suggest that persons who acquired the virus through intravenous drug use or sexual contact should be tested for syphilis. Sexually active persons who are HIV-positive should also be tested. Even if the serologic tests are negative, if the clinical picture suggest syphilis, other methods of diagnosis should be pursued [29].

Treatment of syphilis in the HIV infected patient is undergoing re-evaluation because of the number of treatment failures and cases of neurosyphilis that have been reported in adequately treated persons. Although some experts advise that a treatment regimen appropriate for neurosyphilis be used in early syphilis in HIV infected patients, the CDC currently does not recommend a change in the therapy of early syphilis for these patients [29]. Benzathine penicillin 2.4 million units IM for two doses 7 days apart, or procaine penicillin 4.8 million units IM, is the standard treatment. For penicillin-allergic patients, erythromycin or tetracycline 500 mg orally, four times a day, for 15 days is adequate treatment. If one chooses to treat HIV-positive patients with a regimen appropriate for neurosyphilis, a 10-day course of aqueous penicillin G, 2–4 million units IV, every four hours is the recommended protocol. Regardless of the regimen used, serologic testing after treatment of early syphilis is important for all patients. In patients co-infected with HIV, the CDC recommends quantitative non-treponemal tests every month for the first three months, and at three-month intervals thereafter until a satisfactory serologic response to treatment occurs. An appropriate response is a two-dilution decrease in three months for primary syphilis and in six months for secondary syphilis. If a two-dilution decrease plateaus or an increase in dilution occurs, the patient should be evaluated for the possibility of a treatment failure or re-infection. At this time the cerebrospinal fluid should be examined.

Some studies have been done examining the value of serologic tests in monitoring the response of HIV-positive patients to the treatment of syphilis. Although it appears that the serologic response after treatment is preserved in HIV infected patients classified as CDC group II or III, it is not certain that this will be the case in patients with more advanced disease [30,31].

Gonorrhea

Although infection of the rectum with *N. gonorrhoeae* has been well documented in homosexual men, anorectal ulcerations have been rarely described [31]. Catterall, in 1962, described a patient with a slightly erythematous rectal mucosa and small ulcerations at the anorectal junction [32]. A more recent article suggested that superficial ulcerations and fissures may be associated with rectal gonococcal infections, but do not correlate significantly with positive cultures [33]. There are no cases in the literature to date of anorectal ulcers caused by *N. gonorrhoeae* in a patient with AIDS. However, a high proportion of rectal gonococcal infections are asymptomatic or produce mild symptoms, including constipation, anorectal discomfort, tenesmus, or a mucopurulent discharge [34].

The diagnosis is made by Gram stain and culture of material obtained from rectal swabs or tissue obtained from biopsy. Studies show that the sensitivity of a Gram stain of rectal exudate is higher when obtained through an anoscope [35,36].

Choosing a treatment regimen should be based on the local prevalence of PCN resistant strains, the probability of coexisting STDs, and patient compliance. Treatment for rectal gonococcal infection consists of procaine penicillin G, 4.8 million units IM, plus 1 g probenecid orally. For penicillin-allergic patients, spectinomycin 2 g given as a single IM dose is recommended. Recent studies have shown that ceftriaxone 250 mg given as a single IM dose is more effective against both beta-lactamase-positive and -negative strains of *N. gonorrhoeae* than either penicillin or spectinomycin [37].

Chancroid

Although chancroid is a genital ulcerative disease that is found primarily in Africa and other Third World countries, anorectal manifestations of the disease have been described [38]. The causitive organism is a Gram-negative bacillus, *Hemophilus ducreyi*. After an incubation period of about 3–10 days, an erythematous tender papule develops at the site of inoculation. Over the next couple of days it becomes pustular and ulcerates. These painful ulcers have poorly demarcated borders and a characteristic necrotic irregular base covered by a mucopurulent exudate. There is usually no surrounding induration or erythema. Approximately half of the patients also have painful inguinal lymphadenopathy [39].

The diagnosis is made by culture of material from the ulcer base or enlarged lymph nodes, which is plated on chocolate agar media enriched with vancomycin. A dot-immunobinding serologic test for *H. ducreyi* antibody is also available [40]. Indirect immunoflouresence of ulcer smears using a monoclonal antibody directed against *H. ducreyi* can also be used to make the diagnosis [40,41]. Traditionally *H. ducreyi* has been difficult to isolate and the diagnosis is often made on clinical suspicion and the inability to find other causitive organisms. The availability of DNA probes should greatly facilitate the diagnosis of chancroid [42].

At present, erythromycin 500 mg orally four times per day for 7 days, or ceftriaxone 250 mg IM in a single dose is the treatment of choice. Alternatively, one double-strength tablet of trimethoprim plus sulfamethoxazole twice a day for 7 days or a 1–3 day course of ciprofloxacin 500 mg twice-daily is effective [43]. Scattered reports of resistance to both drugs have appeared, but most ulcers will heal within two weeks. Occasionally, lymph nodes will progress to buboes, even with adequate treatment. This does not imply treatment failure, but the lymph nodes will have to be aspirated (not incised and drained) for healing to occur [39]. No data on the efficacy of treatment in HIV infected patients are available.

Lymphogranuloma venereum

Anorectal involvement with LGV is being reported with increasing frequency in homosexual men [44–46]. It is caused by three specific serotypes of *Chlamydia trachomatis*, L_1, L_2 and L_3. After an incubation period of 3–14 days, a small tender vesicle develops that rapidly ulcerates, becomes painful and then disappears. Unilateral tender erythematous lymphadenopathy will develop 2–3 weeks after the onset of the skin lesions [39]. Systemic symptoms of fever, malaise, hepatitis, meningitis, and conjunctivitis may be associated with this stage of the disease. Rectal involvement is manifested by rectal discharge, perirectal fistulas or abscess, cryptitis, and hematochezia. Progressive rectal strictures, a complication of untreated disease, can occur even in the absence of symptoms. The strictures are generally smooth, circumferential, fixed and firm. In many cases the gross and histologic appearance may be difficult to differentiate from Crohn's disease [47].

C. trachomatis infection can be identified by serologic tests using complement fixation or a microimmunoflourescent assay. However, culture of the organism from the lesions or enlarged lymph nodes remains the 'gold standard' for the diagnosis of LGV [48,49]. The Frei test, which is an intracutaneous injection of antigen prepared from the culture of *Chlamydia* obtained from a bubo, is no longer used.

Tetracycline 500 mg orally four times a day for 2–3 weeks is the treatment of choice for LGV. Other treatment regimens include: doxycycline 100 mg orally twice a day; erythromycin 500 mg orally four times a day; or sulfamethoxazole 1 g orally twice a day. Fluctuant lymph nodes should be aspirated; incision and drainage is not recommended.

Viral infections

Cytomegalovirus

Infection with cytomegalovirus (CMV) is ubiquitous in AIDS patients and can result in many clinical pesentations. At least 95% of homosexual men have antibodies to CMV, with 90% of patients demonstrating active disease [50,51]. Depending on the site and severity of infection and the degree of cellular immunodeficiency, infection may range from an asymptomatic carrier state to a non-specific mononucleosis-like febrile illness, or may develop into a terminal disseminated disease. The virus may be transmitted by saliva, bronchial secretions, contaminated urine, blood transfusions, or sexual contact [52]. Anal genital intercourse is associated with CMV seropositivity.

Among the many manifestations of the disease are gastrointestinal ulcerations. Mucosal ulcers have been documented from the esophagus to the anus. The first case of a small ulcerated anal tumor with 'protozoan-like cells', present in the granulation tissue in the base of the ulcer and in the subendothelial layer of adjacent blood vessels, was reported by Hartz and van de Stadt in 1943 [53]. It has been well documented that CMV can infect any portion of the gastrointestinal tract, and can express itself by inflammation, hemorrhage, ulceration, or perforation [54].

The etiology of gastrointestinal ulcerations is controversial. The accepted theories suggest a progressive vasculitis leading to focal ischemic necrosis and ulcerations [55]. Since CMV is indeed ubiquitous, others have suggested that CMV is just a 'bystander', with other or yet unidentified agents responsible for the ulcerations [56]. Over 70% of homosexual patients with CMV infections also have coexisting alimentary pathogens, so it may be difficult to implicate CMV as the primary cause of these ulcerations [57]. The destruction of the mucosal barrier by trauma or other pathogens may allow entry of CMV into the relatively defenseless submucosal planes. The immunosuppressed state also predisposes the patient to reactivation of latent disease [54].

Anal ulcers secondary to CMV may appear as erythematous patches, with or without punctate ulcerations, or as multiple, deep coalescing ulcers. The ulcer edges are generally smooth and a whitish ulcer membrane may be present (Figs 8.2 and 8.3) [54]. Careful endoscopic examination with multiple biopsies in and around the pathologic sites can successfully establish the diagnosis. Microscopic examination reveals large, basophilic, intranuclear cytomegalic viral inclusions and granular cytoplasmic inclusions which are pathognomonic of the diagnosis. This is seen in endothelial cells, stromal histiocytes and macrophages in the setting of acute and chronic inflammation and ulceration. The basophilic 'smudge-cell' is considered highly

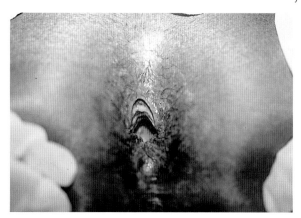

Figure 8.2   Anal ulcer thought secondary to CMV (note proximity of location and broad base).

suggestive of CMV infection [54]. An intense perivascular lymphoplasma-cytic infiltrate, suggestive of a vasculitis, is also frequently seen [58]. His-topathologic examination of biopsy specimens is 92% sensitive in the diagnosis of CMV [59]. Viral culture of rectal swabs is only 30% sensitive. However, in a study on biopsies from autopsy specimens, tissue culture was six times more sensitive than direct histologic examination [60]. Rising antibody titers to CMV antigens in the serum may suggest active CMV infection [61–63]. Immunohistochemical staining by anti-CMV antibodies is a very sensitive method of detecting CMV antigens in tissues. Recently, a probe has become commercially available for the detection of CMV DNA in routinely fixed paraffin-embedded tissues which is even more sensitive than the immunohistochemical tests in AIDS patients [64,65].

Currently, the only treatment for severe CMV infections is 9-(1,3-dihydroxy-2-propoxymethyl) guanine (DHPG; ganciclovir). DHPG is a

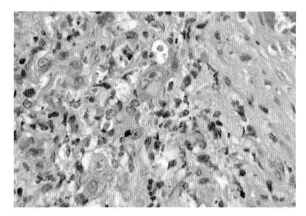

Figure 8.3   Biopsy of ulcer in Plate 8.2 with suggestive 'smudge cells' consistent with CMV.

nucleoside analog of acyclovir, differing by a single hydroxy side chain. This makes the drug approximately 50 times more active against CMV. Intravenous ganciclovir is the only form currently available for clinical use. The usual dosage is 5 mg/kg given twice-daily during initial induction. Maintenance therapy consists of 5–6 mg/kg once-daily or five times per week. Since the drug is renally excreted, the dosage must be adjusted for renal function. Toxic side-effects include severe neutropenia, CNS effects, and gastrointestinal disturbances [66].

Herpes

Herpes simplex virus infections are common in both normal and immu-nocompromised patients. The time between the acquisition of the virus and appearance of the lesions is from 4 to 20 days. Although oral–anal spread has been reported, most cases of anorectal herpes are acquired by anal coitus [67]. Indeed, studies have revealed that over 95% of homosexual men with AIDS have had previous HSV infections [68,69]. Therefore, these patients are susceptible to reactivation and clinical illness.

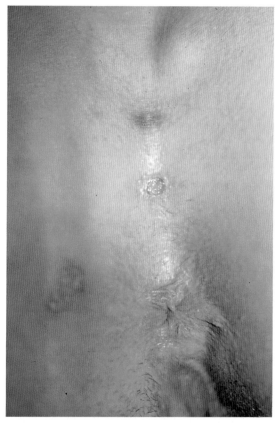

Figure 8.4   Early HSV infection (vesicular) in AIDS patient.

Typically, the illness begins with pruritis, progressing rapidly to severe anal and rectal pain that may radiate to the buttock, groin or thighs. Recurrent perianal lesions in the absence of proctitis is a common finding in AIDS patients. These patients may present with only local pain and itching or pain on defecation. Constitutional symptoms of fever, chills, headache and malaise usually accompany the local symptoms of tenesmus, rectal discharge, constipation, and urinary retention, when proctitis is present. As opposed to immunocompetent persons where recurrent HSV infections are self-limited, persons with AIDS may develop persistent ulcerative lesions [66]. In 1987, the Centres for Disease Control included chronic mucocutaneous HSV infection among the diagnostic criteria for AIDS. Ulcerative HSV infection present for longer than one month in an individual who is HIV-positive or has no other underlying cause of immunodeficiency is diagnostic of AIDS [70]. On physical examination one finds clusters of small vesicles or ulcerations involving the perianal skin, the anal canal, or both (Fig. 8.4). In the immunocompromised patient, however, these ulcera-

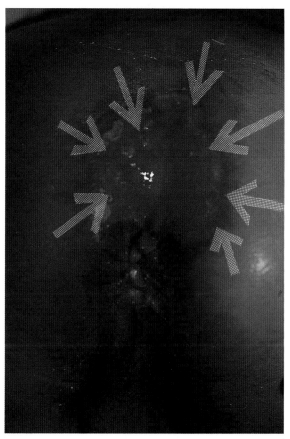

Figure 8.5   Advanced HSV in AIDS patient with large irregular ulceration (arrows) of perianum.

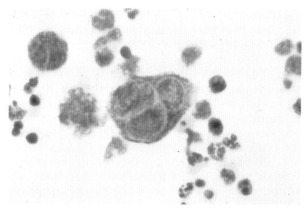

Figure 8.6   Biopsy of HSV ulcer showing multinucleated giant cell.

tions may become confluent and form a large, irregular ulcer surrounded by erythematous, edematous mucosa. These lesions often extend along the gluteal crease to involve the sacrum and may be confused with decubiti ulcers, often delaying the diagnosis (Figs 8.5 and 8.6) [66].

Rectal swabs can be taken, placed immediately in transport media and transported to the laboratory. However, direct tissue culture is more sensitive and should be taken whenever possible. By using the recently available CPE-enhancement techniques, HSV detection is possible within 24 hours in tissue cultures. Tzanck preparation (Wright or Gierinson-stained material from the base of the ulcer) offers a quick, albeit non-specific, method of diagnosis that can be performed in the office. The test is performed by scraping the ulcer base with a wooden spatula or scalpel blade and spreading the material on to a glass slide. The slide is then fixed and stained as if it were a PAP smear. Multinucleated giant cells are seen in both HSV and varicella zoster infections [71]. Skin biopsy is an alternative way of establishing the diagnosis. Cultures and biopsies should be taken from the friable border of the lesions since the central area is usually necrotic or secondarily infected.

Acyclovir has been the cornerstone of treatment of herpetic lesions in normal as well as immunocompromised patients [72–75]. Acyclovir triphosphate acts by selective inhibition of viral DNA polymerase and early termination of DNA chain synthesis. In order to inhibit the growth of HSV, acyclovir requires phosphorylation by a viral thymidine kinase to the monophosphate form, followed by phosphorylation to the active triphosphate form by cellular enzymes. Various routes of administration are available, including topical, oral and intravenous preparations. Topical acyclovir 5% ointment applied to the perianal herpetic lesions six times a day for 7 days accelerates healing. When treated orally, 400 mg five times a day for 7–10 days has been shown to promote healing and shorten viral shedding. For immunocompromised patients with more severe infections, intravenous therapy with 5 mg/kg every 8 hours for 7 days is recommended [72]. There have been increasing reports of acyclovir-resistant herpes simplex virus in normal and immunocompromised patients [76–79]. Any patient with persistent or worsening ulcerations after adequate treatment with acyclovir should have cultures and sensitivities assayed for resistant strains. Most of the acyclovir-resistant strains that have been isolated are thymidine kinase deficient mutants of the virus [80,81]. However, alteration in the substrate specificity of the viral thymidine kinase is an alternative etiology of virus resistance [77,82]. A third mechanism of resistance is selection of viruses with an altered DNA polymerase. Several case reports and one open drug trial have shown promising results using foscarnet to treat acyclovir-resistant HSV. Foscarnet is a direct inhibitor of HSV DNA polymerase and is, therefore, active against thymidine kinase deficient strains [83,84].

Human immunodeficiency virus

Another possible etiologic agent for these pathologic ulcers is the human immunodeficiency virus itself. One of the first clues was the appearance of enveloped virus-like particles, consistent with retrovirus, found by electron microscopy of biopsy specimens from esophageal ulcers [85]. With the use of *in situ* hybridization techniques, HIV has been detected in ulcers from various parts of the gastrointestinal tract [86,87]. Kotler has described deep, chronic ulcers with overhanging edges, throughout the esophagus and colon [88,89]. Morphologically, these ulcers closely resemble the anal lesions that we have seen in our AIDS patients. A study of these anal ulcers using RNA probes for HIV is currently in progress (DK and LG). Identification of the human immunodeficiency virus as an agent in the development or persistence of these refractory ulcers will have important implications for diagnosis and treatment (Figs 8.7 and 8.8).

Cryptococcal infection

Cryptococcosis is an infection caused by the yeast-like fungus *Cryptococcus neoformans*. The prevalence of cryptococcosis in AIDS patients ranges from

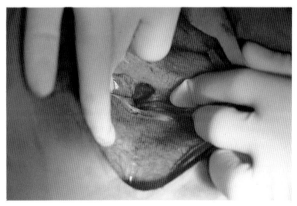

Figure 8.7 'Idiopathic' anal ulcer in HIV-positive patient (note broad clean base extending deep into anal canal).

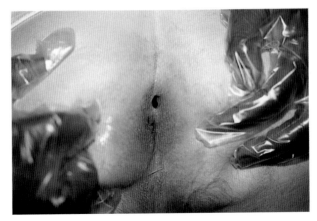

Figure 8.8 'Idiopathic' anal ulcer eroding through perianal skin via the posterior ischiorectal space.

2% to 6% [90,91]. The organism has a predilection for the CNS, but also affects the lungs, bones, skin, GI tract, and may become disseminated. Fungal infections are usually acquired through inhalation of dust containing the fungus or from the droppings of animals infected by it. Traditionally, patients with lymphoma or those receiving high papular lesions, slowly enlarge, and eventually show central softening leading to ulceration [92]. Primary cutaneous infections usually have a good prognosis. However, in AIDS patients the infection can be a result of disseminated disease, making the prognosis more serious. One case of cryptococcal anal ulceration in a patient with AIDS has been described [93]. The patient presented with fever, chills, and hematochezia. On proctoscopy this patient had a large, bloody anal ulcer associated with a fistula. Microscopically, a chronic ulcer with fibroblastic proliferation and many encapsulated yeasts, suggesting *C. neoformans*, were seen. Periodic acid-Schiff, silver stains, and hemotoxylin and eosin stains demonstrated the cryptococci in the microscopic specimen.

Cryptococci are best seen in tissue by staining with methanamine silver or periodic acid-Schiff. Microscopically, the fungus appears as round, yeast-like cells, 4–6 microns in diameter, and surrounded by a large polysac-charide capsule. Sometimes budding forms, indicating active reproduction, may be seen. Serologic tests, by latex agglutination, for cryptococcal antigen in serum and CSF can be helpful in establishing the diagnosis and following the response to therapy [92]. False-positive tests occur occasionally, making culture the definitive diagnostic test. The fungus grows well as smooth, creamy white colonies on Sabouraud's or other simple media at 20–37°C.

A combination of 5-flucytosin, orally, with low-dose intravenous amphotericin B, is active against cryptococcosis. Alternatively, full-dose amphotericin B can be used. Excision of lesions may be sufficient treatment for patients with only a single focus of disease, as seen in the case report. However, it is often the case that patients who are presumed to have only a single focus also have early asymptomatic meningoencephalitis or dis-seminated disease.

Amebiasis

Amebiasis is a protozoan infection caused by *Entamoeba histolytica*. High carrier rates of the parasite have been reported in homosexual men. In the past few years, it has become recognized as a sexually transmitted disease in this population. It is thought that sexual practices such as oral–anal intercourse facilitate transmission of the parasite [94]. Homosexuals with AIDS-related conditions have a very high prevalence of parasitism. Pierce and Abrams studied the prevalence of intestinal parasites in honosexual AIDS patients who had persistent lymphadenopathy syndrome or immune thrombocytopenic purpura: 37% and 41% of patients in each group, respectively, were infected with *E. histolytica*. This is higher than for the homosexual population without AIDS [95].

E. *histolytica* causes a wide range of intestinal diseases, including asymptomatic carriage, acute diarrhea, chronic non-dysenteric colitis, and gastrointestinal ulcerations [96,97]. There is also a great deal of variability between acquisition of the parasite and the onset of symptoms. The vast majority of infections produce only an asymptomatic condition referred to as 'luminal' amebiasis. These are normally healthy persons who have commensal infections, passing only cysts in their stool without clinical symptoms and with negative amebic serology. This must be distinguished from 'invasive' amebiasis, which is the term used for the presence of hematophagous trophozoites in tissue and stool. Invasion of the intestinal wall may be due to the virulence of the organism or host defense factors. Recent studies suggest that the isoenzymes of *E. histolytica* are different between pathogenic and non-pathogenic strains [98]. The isoenzyme patterns in homosexual men indicate a lack of invasive potential [99]. However, it is possible that non-invasive strains may elicit a pathogenic response in patients who are immunologically compromised or who have prolonged contact of the parasite with the host tissue. Mirelman has also reported that the isoenzyme patterns of non-invasive isolates can be converted to patterns that make them pathogenic by culturing them with different intestinal flora [100]. Thus, the polymicrobial nature of the gastrointestinal tract of homosexual AIDS patients may further enhance the pathogenicity of the parasite.

On proctoscopy, these lesions appear as flask-shaped ulcers with undermined edges and a fairly clean base. Early lesions may be covered with a yellow, raised exudate. As the ulcer extends, the crater may be filled with necrotic tissue. The definitive diagnosis, however, is made by identification of the cysts or trophozoites of *E. histolytica* in stool samples, aspirates or biopsy specimens from mucosal lesions. Seroepidemiologic studies have recently shown that a one-time stool examination for cysts identifies only 20–40% of infections in high-risk groups [101]. Serologic testing for anti-amebic antibodies with radioimmunoassay or counterimmunoelectrophoresis can also be helpful [102].

Appropriate drug therapy is key in the management of intestinal amebiasis. The treatment of choice is metronidazole 750 mg orally three times a day for 5–10 days. Recent evaluation of the therapeutic efficacy of paromomycin in the treatment of endemic amebiasis in homosexual men has shown promising results [103]. A luminal amebicide can also be used, especially in chronic intestinal infections. These drugs include diloxanide and iodoquinol (650 mg orally three times a day for 20 days). Intestinal amebiasis commonly recurs, even though the host has not been reinfected. Therefore close follow-up for several months is mandatory. Arguments have raged over whether or not to treat AIDS patients who are asymptomatic carriers of the parasite. Although the study by Allison-Jones showed no increase in GI symptoms in homosexual men with the parasite as compared with uninfected controls, others argue that 'non-pathogenic' *E. histolytica* infections in homosexual man may cause disease [98,104]. Since amebiasis is a sexually transmitted disease in this population, it should be treated as such. Therefore, asymptomatic carriers should be treated.

Idiopathic lesions

Recently in the literature there have been reports of severe aphthous ulcerations that respond to local or systemic steroid therapy [105,106]. Although most report ulcers involving the mouth and esophagus, similar ulcers have also been found in the colon. Biopsy specimens from these lesions did not show the presence of virus or fungus, and the conditions responded rapidly to high-dose prednisone therapy [107]. We have found similar non-specific anal ulcerations associated with HIV infection that have improved with 80 mg/cm^3 of depomerial intralesional injection.

Trauma

A wide range of foreign objects are introduced into the anus by accident, for erotic purposes, for self-treatment, or by assault. Vibrators, bottles, fists and even anal coitus may cause tears and fissures in the anal mucosa. Traumatic fissures are usually related to a specific event and are associated with rectal pain and bleeding. It is important to obtain a candid history of specific sexual activities, past history of anorectal problems and sexually transmitted diseases. Abdominal examination and x-rays are used to exclude signs of peritonitis, pneumoperitoneum and retained foreign bodies. An acute abdomen is an indication for prompt surgical intervention. Rectal examination and sigmoidoscopy usually reveal a superficial laceration. Although most fissures will stop bleeding spontaneously, electrocautery may be needed to stop persistent bleeding. When it is clear that there is no infectious or neoplastic etiology for the ulcer, conservative management with Sitz baths, bulk laxatives, analgesics and instructions for abstinence from anal intercourse is the treatment of choice. On rare occasions, one may see varying degrees of disruption of the anal sphincter. For acute injuries with minimal inflammation, primary repair of the internal sphincter under local anesthesia in the operating room is recommended. When the wound is infected, it should be left open, presacral drainage established, and a diverting end colostomy with mucus fistula created [108–111].

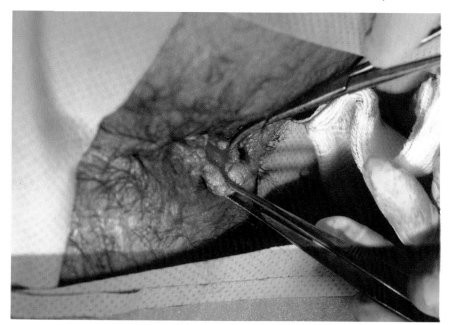

Figure 8.9 Kaposi's sarcoma in fissure in AIDS patient.

Neoplasia

Increasing numbers of AIDS patients are afflicted by a variety of neoplastic disorders related to their immunocompromised state [112–121]. These malignant anorectal diseases may present as anal strictures, warts, fungating masses, fissures and ulcers. Kaposi's sarcoma (Fig. 8.9), non-Hodgkin's lymphoma (Fig. 8.10) and cloacogenic or squamous cell carcinoma (Fig. 8.11) are the most common tumours identified in biopsies of anal ulcers. With the increasing prevalence of these neoplastic lesions, we recommend incisional

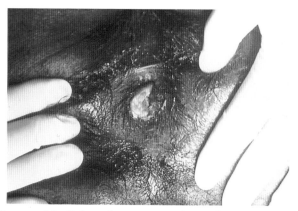

Figure 8.10 Immunoblastic lymphoma presenting as fissures in AIDS patient.

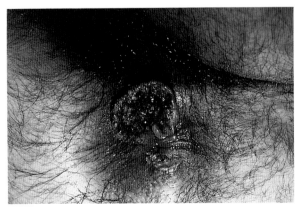

Figure 8.11   Squamous cell carcinoma presenting as ulcer in AIDS patient.

biopsy of all anorectal ulcers in this high-risk group. For further information about these malignancies, refer to Chapter 11.

Summary

There is mounting evidence showing a clear association between genital ulcerations and the human immunodeficiency virus. Therefore, the surgeon must have a high index of suspicion in managing any atypical ulcer in this high-risk population. A thorough and candid history of sexual practices, anorectal trauma, previous operations, coexistent medical problems, and, especially, active or quiescent venereal diseases is imperative. It is important to distinguish between the sharp pain on defecation associated with the more benign fissures, and deeper pelvic pain, associated with supporation and bleeding, suggesting a more pathologic process. In addition, determining the extent of diarrhea is necessary prior to selecting an appropriate operative procedure, so as not to compromise sphincter function in patients prone to life-long diarrhea.

On presentation to the clinic, many of these patients are *in extremis* and the physical examination may be limited. It is important to ascertain the location of the fissure and a sense of the basal sphincter tone to help differentiate pathologic from benign fissures. Bridging sentinal tags, sometimes seen in inflammatory bowel disease, also herald pathologic fissures. In addition, the viral-induced fissures tend to occur somewhat more proximally in the anal canal. Initially, they dissect submucosally along the superficial aspects of the internal sphincter as it courses proximally, then either burrow through the internal anal sphincter or underneath it at its most distal point. Many times one can see a reservoir of pus or feces in the crater of the ulcer as the disease progresses. We feel it is necessary to examine all patients under anesthesia. At that time, the anal canal can be more adequately assessed and tissue samples can be taken for further diagnostic tests.

In addition to a comprehensive physical examination, the work-up should include: (1) a serologic tests for syphilis, (2) dark-field examination of the ulcer exudate, (3) a PPD and energy panel, (4) examination of stool for ova and parasites, (5) tissue from the sides and base of the ulcer for Gram's stain and culture with antibiotic sensitivities for *H. ducreyi*, herpes simplex, *N. gonorrhoeae*, tuberculosis and CMV, (6) a biopsy specimen for histologic examination including special stains for acid-fast bacilli, fungi, and spirochetes, and (7) complement fixation for *Chlamydia trachomatis*.

The treatment approach will depend on the etiology of the ulcer, as well as the patient's immunologic status and underlying medical problems. If the fissure appears benign, a lateral internal sphincterotomy may be performed with an open technique. More conservative management, including Sitz baths, bulk-producing agents and a topical anesthetic, can be used for these fissures as well as those associated with a traumatic etiology. For those patients with a clear infectious etiology, the appropriate chemotherapeutic regimen should be promptly instituted. In addition, a significant number of these patients will benefit from surgical debridement of the ulcer. Any pocketing should be widely opened (usually involving a partial internal sphincterotomy) to allow adequate drainage of the pocket and avoid the pain associated with collection of feces or pus. For those ulcers with no known traumatic, infectious or neoplastic etiology, we have empirically injected the base of these ulcers with Depomedrol ($80\,mg/cm^3$) every two weeks. We have been encouraged by the short-term results and pain control. As these ulcers continue, they may lead to erosion of the inferior hemorrhoidal vessels and nerves and cause debilitating pain or life-threatening hemorrhage. In this case, nothing short of suture ligation of the ulcer with concomitant end sigmoid colectomy will abate this complication.

References

1. Pepin J, Plummer FA, Brunham RC, Piot P, Cameron DW, Ronald AR. The interaction of HIV infection and other sexually transmitted diseases: an opportunity for intervention. *AIDS* 1939; **3**:3–9.
2. O'Farrell N. Transmission of HIV: genital ulceration, sexual behavior, and circumcision. *Lancet* 1989; **ii**:1157.
3. Stamm WE, Handsfield HH, Rompalo AM, Ashley RL, Roberts PL, Corey L. The association between genital ulcer disease and aquisition of HIV infection in homosexual men. *JAMA* 1988; **260**:1429–33.
4. Notaras MJ. Anal fissure and stenosis. In *Surgical Clinics of North America: Techniques of Colorectal Surgery*, 1988; **68**:1427–40.
5. Northmann BJ, Schuster MM. Internal anal sphincter derangement with anal fissures. *Gastroenterology* 1974; **67**:216–20.
6. Hancock BD. The internal sphincter and anal fissure. *Br J Surg* 1977; **64**:92–5.
7. Gibbons CP, Read NW. Anal hypertonia in fissures: cause or effect? *Br J Surg* 1986; **73**:443–5.
8. Khubchandani IT, Reed JF. Sequelae of internal sphincterotomy for chronic fissure-in-ano. *Br J Surg* 1989;**76**:431–4.
9. Chowcat NL, Araujo JG, Boulos PB. Internal sphincterotomy for chronic anal fissure: long term effects on anal pressure. *Br J Surg* 1986; **73**:915–16.
10. Cerdan FJ, Ruiz de Leon A, Azpiroz F, *et al*. Anal sphincter pressure in fissure-

in-ano before and after lateral internal sphincterotomy. *Dis Colon Rectum* 1982; **25**:198–201.

11. Elam AL, Ray VG. Sexually related trauma: a review. *Ann Emerg Med* 1986; **15**:576–84.
12. Centers for Disease Control. Tuberculosis provisional data—United States 1986. *MMWR* 1987; **36**:254–55.
13. Centers for Disease Control. Tuberculosis and the aquired immunodeficiency syndrome—Florida. *MMWR* 1986; **35**:587–90.
14. Farer LS, Snider DE. Tuberculosis: current recommendations for cure and control. *Postgrad Med* 1988; **84**(1):58–73.
15. Nunn PP, McAdam PKWJ. Mycobacterial infections and AIDS. *Br Med Bull* 1988; **44**(3):801–13.
16. Chaisson RE, Schecter GF, Theuer CP, *et al*. Tuberculosis in patients with the aquired immunodeficiency syndrome: clinical features, response to therapy, and survival. *Am Rev Resp Dis* 1987; **136**:570–4.
17. Pitchenik AE, Cole C, Russell BW, *et al*. Tuberculosis, atypical mycobacteriosis, and the aquired immunodeficiency syndrome among Haitian and non-Haitian patients in south Florida. *Ann Inter Med* 1984; **101**:641–5.
18. Dean ED, Cabanas DK, Daly WJ, *et al*. Mycobacterium tuberculosis. Direct rapid detection of the complex in sputum by DNA probe assay. Interscience Conference on Antimicrobial Agents and Chemotherapy, 1987. Abstract 1355; 332.
19. Centers for Disease Control. Continuing increase in infectious syphilis—United States. *MMWR* 1988; **37**:35–8.
20. Centers for Disease Control. Syphilis and congenital syphilis—United States: 1985–1988. *MMWR* 1988; **37**:486–9.
21. Potterat JJ. Does syphilis fascilitate sexual aquisition of HIV? *JAMA* 1987; **258**:473–4.
22. Jaffe HW. The laboratory diagnosis of syphilis. *Ann Intern Med* 1975; **83**:846–50.
23. Freinkel AL. Histological aspects of sexually transmitted genital lesions. *Histopath* 1987; **11**:819–31.
24. Al-Samairai HT, Henderson WG. Immunoflourescent staining of *T. pallidum* and *T. pectinue* in tissue fixed in formalin and embedded in paraffin wax. *Br J Ven Dis* 1977; **53**:1–11.
25. Becket JH, Bigbee MA. Immunoperoxidase localization of *T. pallidum*. *Arch Pathol Lab Med* 1979; **103**:135–8.
26. Schultz S, Araneta MRG, Joseph SC. Neurosyphilis and HIV infection. *New Engl J Med* 1987; **317**:1474.
27. Hicks CB, Benson PM, Lupton GP, Tramont EC. Seronegative secondary syphilis in a patient infected with the aquired immunodeficiency virus (HIV) with Kaposi's sarcoma: a diagnostic dilemma. *Ann Intern Med* 1987; **107**:492–4.
28. Anonymous. Leads from the MMWR: Recommendations for diagnosing and treating syphilis in HIV-infected patients. *JAMA* 1988; **260**(17):2488–9.
29. Terry PM, Page ML, Goldmeier D. Are serologic tests of value in diagnosing and monitoring response to treatment of syphilis in patients infected with human immunodeficiency virus? *Genitourin Med* 1988; **64**:219–22.
30. Centers for Disease Control. Classification system for human T-lymphotrophic virus type III/lyphadenopathy-associated virus infections. *MMWR* 1986; **35**:334–9.
31. Harkness AH. The pathology of gonorrhoea. *Br J Vener Dis* 1948;**24**:137.
32. Catterall RR. Anorectal gonorrhoea. *Proc R Soc Med* 1962; **55**:871.
33. Lebedeff DA, Hochman EB. Rectal gonorrhea in men: diagnosis and treatment. *Ann Intern Med* 1980; **92**:463–6.

34. Pariser H, Marino AF. Gonorrhea: frequency of unrecognized reservoirs. *South Med J* 1970; **63**:198–202.
35. Deheragoda P., Diagnosis of anorectal gonorrhoea by blind anorectal swabs compared with direct vision swabs taken via a proctoscope. *Br J Vener Dis* 1977; **53**:311–14.
36. William DC, Felman YM, Riccardi NB. The utility of anoscopy in the rapid diagnosis of symptomatic anorectal gonorrhea in men. *Sex Trans Dis* 1981; **8**:16–19.
37. Judson FN, Ehret JM, Handsfield HH. Comparative study of ceftriaxone and spectinomycin for treatment of pharyngeal and anorectal gonorrhea. *JAMA* 1985; **253**:1417–19.
38. Carman ML. *Colon and Rectal Surgery*. Philadelphia: Lippincott, 1984.
39. Levin S, Pottage JC, Kessler HA, Benson CA, Goodman, Trenholme GM. Genital ulcers and lymphadenopathy. *DM* 1987; April: 200–2.
40. Schalla WO, Sanders LL, Schmid GP, Tam MR, Morse SA. Use of dot-immunobinding and immunoflourescence assays to investigate clinically suspected cases of chancroid. *J Infect Dis* 1986; **153**:879–87.
41. Museyi K, Van Dyck E, Vervoort T, Taylor D, Hoge C, Piot P. Use of an enzyme immunoassay to detect serum IgG antibodies to *Haemophilus ducreyi*. *J Infect Dis* 1988; **157**:1039–43.
42. Parsons LM, Shayegani M, Waring AL, Bopp LH. DNA probes for the identification of *Haemophilus ducreyi*. *J Clin Microbiol* 1989; **27**:1441–5.
43. Boyd AS. Clinical efficacy of antimicrobial therapy in *Haemophilus ducreyi* infections. *Arch Dermatol* 1989; **125**:1399–405.
44. Palmer WL, Kirsner JB, Rodaniche EC. Studies on *lymphogranuloma venereum* infections of the rectum. *Jama* 1942; **118**:517.
45. Levine JS, Smith PD, Brugge WR. Chronic proctitis in male homosexuals due to *lymphogranuloma venereum*. *Gastroenterology* 1980; **79**:563–5.
46. Quinn TC, Goodell SE, Mkhitichian PAC, *et al*. *Chlamydia trachomatis* proctitis. *New Engl J Med* 1981; **305**:195–200.
47. Neimark S. Venereal diseases of the intestine. In Berk JE, Haubrich WS, Kalser MH, Roth JLA, Schaffner F (eds), *Bockus Gastroenterology*. New York: WB Saunders, 1985, 2037–55.
48. Spence MR. The treatment of gonorrhea, syphilis, chancroid, lymphogranuloma venereum and granuloma inguinale. *Clin Obs Gynecol* 1988; **31**:453–65.
49. Goldmeier D, Darougar S. Isolation of *Chlamydia trachomatis* from throat and rectum of homosexual men. *Br J Vener Dis* 1977; **53**:184–5.
50. Lange M, Klein EB, Kornfield H, Cooper LZ, Grieco MH. Cytomegalovirus isolation from healthy homosexual men. *JAMA* 1984; **252**:1908–10.
51. Drew WL, Mintz L, Miner RC, Sands M, Ketterer B. Prevalence of cytomegalovirus infection in homosexual men. *J Infect Dis* 1981; **143**:188–92.
52. Balthazar EJ, Megibow AJ, Hulnick DH. Cytomegalovirus esohagitis and gastritis in AIDS. *AJR* 1985; **144**:1201–4.
53. Hartz PH, van de Stadt PF. The occurrence of protozoan-like cells in a biopsy from the anus. *Am J Clin Pathol* 1943; **13**:148.
54. Wexner SD, Smith WB, Trillo C, Hopkins BS, Dailey TH. Emergency colectomy for CMV ileocolitis in patients with the aquired immunodeficiency syndrome. *Dis Col Rec* 1988; **31**:755–61.
55. Frank D, Raicht R. Intestinal perforation associated with cytomegalovirus infection in patients with aquired immunodeficiency syndrome. *Am J Gastroenterol* 1984; **79**:201–5.
56. Goodman ZD, Boitnott JK, Yardley JH. Perforation of the colon associated with cytomegalovirus infection *Dig. Dis Sci* 1979; **24**: 376–80.

57. Hinnant HL, Rotterdam HZ, Bell ET, Tapper ML. Cytomagalovirus infection of the alimentary tract: a clinicopathologic correlation. *Am J Gastroenterol* 1986; **81**:944–50.
58. DeRiso AJ, Kemeny MM. Torres RA, Oliver JM. Multiple jejunal perforations secondary to cytomegalovirus in a patient with aquired immunodeficiency syndrome: case report and review. *Dig Dis Sci* 1989; **34**:623–9.
59. Culpepper-Morgan JA, Kotler DP, Scholes JV, Tierney AR. Evaluation of diagnostic criteria for mucosal cytomegalic inclusion disease in the aquired immunodeficiency syndrome. *Am J Gastroenterol* 1987; **82**:1264–70.
60. Smith TF, Holley KE, Keys TF, Wascaget FF. Cytomegalovirus studies of autopsy tissue. I: Virus isolation. *Am J Clin Pathol* 1975; **63**:854.
61. Kangro HO, Griffiths PD, Huber HJ, Heath RB. Specific IgM class antibody production following infection with cytomegalovirus. *J. Med Virol* 1982; **10**:203–12.
62. Dylewski, J, Chon S, Merigan TC. Absence of detectable IgM antibody during cytomegalovirus disease in patients with AIDS. *New Engl J Med* 1983; **309**:493.
63. Panjwani DD, Ball NG, Berry NJ. Virologic and serologic diagnosis of CMV infection in bone marrow allograft recipients. *J Med Virol* 1985; **16**:357–65.
64. Keh WC, Gerber MA. *In situ* hybridization for cytomegalovirus DNA in AIDS patients. *Am J Pathol* 1988; **131**:490–6.
65. Unger ER, Budgeon LR, Myerson D, Brigati DJ. Viral diagnosis by *in situ* hybridization: description of a rapid simplified colorimetric method. *Am J Surg Pathol* 1986; **10**:1–8.
66. Drew WL, Buhles W, Erlick KS. Herpesvirus infections (cytomegalovirus, herpes simplex virus, varicella-zoster virus): how to use gangciclovir (DHPG) and acyclovir. *Inf Dis Clinics NA* 1988; **2**: 495–509.
67. Jacobs E. Anal infections caused by herpes simplex virus. *Dis Col Rec* 1976; **19**:151–7.
68. Nerurkar L, Goedert J, Wallen W, *et al*. Study of antiviral antibodies in sera of homosexual men. *J Fed Proc* 1983; **42**:6109.
69. Rogers MF, Morens DM, Stewart JA, *et al*. National case control study of Kaposi's sarcoma and *Pneumocystis carinii* pneumonia in homosexual men. 2: Laboratory results. *Ann Intern Med* 1983; **99**:151–8.
70. Revision of the CDC surveillance case definition for acquired immunodeficiency syndrome. *MMWR* 1987; **36** (Suppl): 1s-15s.
71. Feder HM, Renfro L, Schmidt DD. Common questions about herpes simplex. *Hosp Prac* 1989; 30 Jan: 50–62.
72. Gold D, Corey L. Acyclovir prophylaxis for herpes simplex virus infection. *Antimicrob Agents Chemother* 1987; **31**:361–7.
73. Strauss SE, Smith HA, Brickman C, *et al*. Acyclovir for chronic mucocutaneous herpes simplex virus infection in immunosuppressed patients. *Ann Intern Med* 1982; **96**:270–7.
74. Dorsky DI, Crumpacker CS. Drugs five years later: acyclovir. *Ann Intern Med* 1987; **107**:859–74.
75. Whitley RJ, Levin M, Barton N, *et al*. Infections caused by herpes simplex virus in the immunocompromised host: natural history and topical acyclovir therapy. *J Infect Dis* 1984; **150**:323–9.
76. Erlich KS, Mills J, Chatis P, *et al*. Acyclovir-resistant herpes simplex virus infections in patients with the acquired immunodeficiency syndrome. *New Engl J Med* 1989; **320**:293–6.
77. Ellis MN, Keller PM, Fyfe JA, *et al*. Clinical isolate of herpes simplex type-2 that induces a thymidine kinase with altered substrate specificity. *Antimicrob Agents Chemother* 1987; **31**:1117–25.
78. Svennerholm B, Vahlne A, Lowhagen GB, *et al*. Sensitivity of HSV strains

isolated before and after treatment with acyclovir. *Scand J Infect Dis* 1985; **47** (Suppl): 149–54.

79. Schenazi RF, delBene V, Scott RT. Characterization of acyclovir-resistant and -sensitive herpes simpex virus isolated from a patient with an aquired immune deficiency. *J. Antimicrob Chemother* 1986; **18** (Suppl B):127–34.

80. Schnipper LE, Crumpacker CS. Resistance of herpes simplex virus to acycloguanosine: role of viral thymidine kinase and DNA polymerase loci. *Proc Natl Acad Sci USA* 1980; **77**:2270–3.

81. Barry DW, Lehrman SN, Ellis MN. Clinical and laboratory experience with acyclovir-resistant herpes virus. *J Antimicrob Chemother* 1986; **18**(Suppl B): 75–84.

82. Darby G, Field HJ, Salisbury SA. Altered substrate specificity of herpes simplex virus thymidine kinase confers acyclovir-resistance. *Nature* 1981; **289**:81–3.

83. Youle MM, Hawkins DA, Collins P, *et al*. Acyclovir-resistant herpes in AIDS treated with foscarnet (letter). *Lancet* 1988; 6 Aug: 341–2.

84. Erlich KS, Jacobson MA, Koehler JE, *et al*. Foscarnet therapy for severe acyclovir-resistant herpes simplex virus type-2 infections in patients with the acquired immunodeficiency syndrome (AIDS). *Ann Intern Med* 1989; **110**:710–13.

85. Rabeneck L, Boyko WJ, McLean DM, *et al*. Unusual esophageal ulcers containing enveloped-virus like particles in homosexual men. *Gastroenterology* 1986; **90**:1882–9.

86. Nelson JA, Wiley CA, Reynolds-Kohler C, *et al*. Human immunodeficiency virus detected in bowel epithelium from patients with gastrointestinal symptoms. *Lancet* 1988; **1**:259–62.

87. Levy JA, Margaretten W, Nelson J. Detection of HIV in enterochromaffin cells in the rectal mucosa of an AIDS patient. *Am J Gastroenterol* 1989; **84**:787–9.

88. Fox CH, Kotler DP, Tierney A, Wilson CS, Fauci AS. Detection of HIV-1 RNA in the lamina propria of patients with AIDS and gastrointestinal disease. *J Infect Dis* 1989; **159**:467–71.

89. Kotler DP, Wilson CS, Haroutiourian G, Fox CH. Detection of human immunodeficiency virus-1 by ^{35}S-RNA *in situ* hybridization in solitary esophageal ulcers in two patients with the acquired immunodeficiency syndrome. *Am J Gastroenterol* 1989; **84**:313–17.

90. Kovacs J, Kovacs A, Polis M, *et al*. Cryptococcosis in the acquired immunodeficiency syndrome. *Ann Intern Med* 1985; **103**:533–8.

91. Zuger A, Louie E, Holzmann R, *et al*. Cryptococcal disease in patients with the acquired immunodeficiency syndrome. *Ann Intern Med* 1986; **104**:234–40.

92. Bennett JE. The deep mycoses. In Petersdorf RG, Adams RD, Braunwald E, Isselbacher KJ, Martin JB, Wilson JD (eds), *Harrison's Principles of Internal Medicine*. New York: McGraw-Hill, 1983:1056–7.

93. VanCalck M, Motte S, Rickaert F, *et al*. Cryptococcal anal ulceration in a patient with AIDS. *Am J Gastroenterol* 1988; **83**:1306–8.

94. Phillips SC, Mildvan D, William DC, Gelb AM, White MC. Sexual transmission of enteric protozoa and helminths in a venereal disease clinic population. *New Engl J Med* 1981; **305**:603–6.

95. Pearce RB, Abrahms DI. *Entamoeba histolytica* in homosexual men. *New Engl J Med* 1987; **316**(11):691–2.

96. Wanke C, Butler T, Islam M. Epidemiologic and clinical features of invasive amebiasis in Bangladesh: a case-control comparison with other diarrheal diseases and postmortem finding. *Am J Trop Med Hyg* 1988; **38**:335–41.

97. Davidson BR, Neoptalemos JP, Watkin D, Talbot TC. Invasive amoebiasis an unusual presentation. *Gut* 1988; **29**:682–5.

98. Krogstad DJ. Isoenzyme patterns and pathogenicity in amoebic infection. *New Engl J Med* 1986; **315**:390–1.
99. Allason-Jones E, Mindel A, Sargeaunt P, Williams P. *Entamoeba histolytica* as a commensal intestinal parasite in homosexual men. *New Engl J Med* 1986; **315**:353–6.
100. Mirelman D, Bracha R, Chayen A, Aust-Kettis A, Diamond LS. *Entamoeba histolytica*: effects of growth conditions and bacterial associates on isoenzyme patterns and virulence. *Exp Parasitol* 1986; **62**:142–8.
101. Holtan N. Amebiasis: the ancient scourge is still with us. *Postgrad Med* 1988; **83**:65–72.
102. Pillai S, Mohimen A. A solid-phase sandwich radioimmunoassay for *Entamoeba histolytica* proteins and the detection of circulating antigens in amoebiasis. *Gastroenterology* 1982; **83**:1210–6.
103. Sullam PH, Slutkin G, Gottlieb AB, Mills J. Paromomycin therapy of endemic amebiasis in homosexual men. *Sex Trans Dis* 1986; **13**:151–5.
104. Petri WA, Ravdin JI. Treatment of homosexual men infected with *Entamoeba histolytica*. *New Engl J Med* 1986; **315**(6):393.
105. Bach MC, Valenti AJ, Howell DA, Smith TJ. Odynophagia form aphthous ulcers of the pharynx and esophagus in the acquired immunodeficiency syndrome. *Ann Intern Med* 1988; **109**:338–9.
106. Dretler RH, Raucher DB. Giant esophageal ulcer healed with steroid therapy in an AIDS patient. *Rev Infect Dis* 1989; **11**:768–9.
107. Bach MC, Howell DA, Valenti AJ, *et al.* Aphthous ulcerations of the gastro-intestinal tract in patients with acquired immunodeficiency syndrome (AIDS). *Ann Intern Med* 1990; **112**:465–7.
108. Barone JE, Yee J, Nealson TF. Management of foreign bodies and trauma of the rectum. *Surg Gynecol Obstet* 1983; **156**:453–7.
109. Grasberger RC, Hirsch EF. Rectal trauma—a retrospective analysis and guidelines for therapy. *Am J Surg* 1983; **145**:795–9.
110. Haas PA, Fox TA. Civilian injuries of the rectum and anus. *Dis Col Rec* 1979; **22**:17–23.
111. Schiff AF. Examination and treatment of a male rape victim. *South Med J* 1980; **73**:1498–502.
112. Nash G, Allen W, Nash S. Atypical lesions of the anal mucosa in homosexual men. *JAMA* 1986; **256**(7):873–6.
113. Frazer IH, Crapper RM, Medley G, Brown TC, Mackay IR. Association between anorectal dysplasia, human papillomavirus, and human immunodeficiency virus infection in homosexual men. *Lancet* 1986; 20 Sept: 657–60.
114. Rudlinger R, Buchmann P. HPV 16-positive bowenoid papulosis and squamous-cells carcinoma of the anus in an HIV-positive man. *Dis Col Rec* 1989; **32**:1042–5.
115. Cooper HS, Patchefsky AS, Marks G. Cloacogenic carcinoma of the anorectum in homosexual men: an observation of four cases. *Dis Col Rec* 1979; **22**:557–8.
116. Lee MH, Waxman M, Gillooley JF. Primary malignant lymphoma of the anorectum in homosexual men. *Dis Col Rec* 1986; **29**:413–16.
117. Burkes RL, Meyer PR, Gill PS, Parker JW, Rasheed S, Levine AM. Rectal lymphoma in homosexual men. *Arch Intern Med* 1986; **146**:913–15.
118. Mehta K, Pawel BR. Human immunodeficiency virus-associated large-cell immunoblastic lymphoma presenting as a perianal abscess. *Arch Pathol Lab Med* 1989; **113**:531–3.
119. Morrison JG, Scharfenberg, JC, Timmcke AE. Perianal lymphoma as a manifestation of the acquired immune deficiency syndrome. *Dis Col Rec* 1989; **32**:521–3.

120. Endean ED, Ross CW, Strodel WE. Kaposi's sarcoma appearing as a rectal ulcer. *Surgery* 1987; **101**:767–9.
121. Grody WW, Lewin KJ, Naeim F. Detection of cytomegalovirus DNA in classic and epidemic Kaposi's sarcoma by *in situ* hybridization. *Human Pathol* 1988; **19**:524–8.

9

Anal and perianal sepsis
Bruce S Gingold

Introduction

Under normal circumstances, the rectum and anus are practically impervious to infection. When one considers the billions of bacteria and their byproducts that pass through this part of the body every day, and when one realizes that microscopic breaks in the mucosa occur constantly owing to the mechanical nature of the act of defecation, it is quite remarkable that anal and perianal sepsis is not a constant condition. For many years it has been well-known that factors interfering with the normal body defenses could result in significant breakdowns in this area. Patients with leukemia, those on steroids and patients with transplants, especially prior to the development of cyclosporin and other current antirejection medications, have had frequent problems in this area; and, in fact, perianal breakdown has been a frequent cause of death in this patient population. Since 1981, with the first description of immunocompromised patients infected with the human immunodeficiency virus [1], this pattern is being repeated.

Up to December 1989, approximately 100 000 Americans had been diagnosed as having AIDS. It is estimated that an additional 1.5 million people have been infected by this virus. Between 2% and 9% of HIV-positive patients develop AIDS each year [2]. As the number of patients with full-blown AIDS increases, the number of individuals with serious anal and perianal infections are expected to increase dramatically. Since immunocompromised patients do not have the same healing characteristics as uninfected patients, surgeons in general and colorectal surgeons in particular will have to appreciate the resulting increased mortality and morbidity, and so develop new strategies to minimize the risks of surgery in affected patients, as well as the risks to medical personnel responsible for their care.

General principles

The human immunodeficiency virus is an RNA retrovirus which selectively attacks the T4 (helper) lymphocytes by binding the T4 cellular antigen with the major envelope glycoprotein GP120 [2]. As the T4 population is reduced, the body becomes susceptible to opportunistic infections and malignant neoplasms. It is these factors that result in the approximately 50% mortality

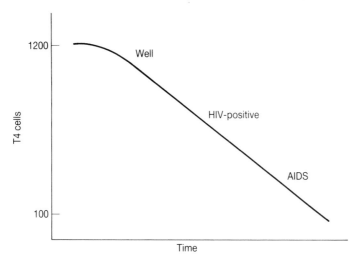

Figure 9.1   Relationship of T4 cell population to the development of AIDS.

at present of all patients who have developed AIDS. With time, it is anticipated that the mortality will approach 100% [3].

Patients infected with HIV do not always present with AIDS. There is a progression from initial exposure to the virus, to seroconversion (HIV-positive), to AIDS (Fig. 9.1). This appears to correlate with the number of surviving T4 lymphocytes in the infected patient. It is the feeling of the author that the risk of postoperative complications will in large part be determined by the number of functioning T cells in the patient. This is by no means the only significant factor, of course, since other factors such as total white blood cell count, nutritional status and an intact blood clotting mechanism must be considered.

While a review of the literature does not reveal any prospective studies to date that prove a direct relationship with the paucity of T4 cells and the likelihood of postoperative complications, it seems reasonable to assume this is a significant factor, and it is suggested that any HIV-positive patient who is to undergo elective surgery of any kind has a preoperative evaluation including total lymphocyte count, total T4 count, T4/T8 ratio, white blood count and serum albumin and total protein. In certain cases the risk of morbidity, including poor wound healing, sepsis, etc., may make it advisable to minimize operative procedures and, in extreme cases, to avoid non-essential elective surgery entirely, especially if the T4 count is below 100.

Another aspect that must be considered is the exposure risks to operating room personnel. At present, the CDC estimates that the risk of seroconversion following needlestick injuries from HIV-positive patients is 0.5% [4]. The American College of Surgeons places this risk at 0.13–0.39% [5]. By developing and practicing 'safe surgery' techniques the number of these types of injuries may be reduced.

Abscesses and fistulae-in-ano

In the HIV-negative patient it is felt that almost all anorectal abscesses begin as infections of the anal glands [6]. The infectious process then extends to a specific rectal space. When the abscess ruptures through the skin or is incised, a fistula-in-ano is established. Hanley drew up a classification of abscesses based on anatomical location (Table 9.1) [7].

Parks [8] divided fistulae-in-ano into four types based on his experience with 400 patients: *intrasphincteric* (type 1), in which the fistula reaches only the intrasphincteric plane (Fig. 9.2A); *transsphincteric* (type 2), where the tract passes from the intrasphincteric plane through the external sphincter mechanism into the ischiorectal space and out the skin (Fig. 9.2B); *suprasphincteric* (type 3), in which the tract passes in the intersphincteric plane over the top of the puborectalis then downward through the levator ani musculature into the ischiorectal fossa and eventually to the skin (Fig. 9.2C); and *extrasphincteric* (type 4), where the tract passes from the perineal skin through the ischiorectal space and levator muscles into the rectum above the puborectalis sling (Fig. 9.2D). The latter tract is outside the external sphincter complex altogether and is quite difficult to treat. Since rectal pressure is higher than atmospheric pressure, extrasphincteric fistulae do not resolve spontaneously and may require diverting colostomy to achieve healing. Closure of the internal opening by suturing [6] and by a mucosal advancement flap technique have been described for complex fistulae-in-ano (in immunocompetent patients) with promising results [9]. Fortunately type 4 fistula-in-ano is relatively rare. It was found in only 5% of Parks' series, while type 1 was seen in 45%, type 2 in 30%, and type 3 in 20%. These percentages of course deal with immunocompetent patients for the most part, since the article was written in the pre-AIDS era. Ischiorectal abscesses and fistula-in-ano are extremely common in HIV-positive patients, espe-

Table 9.1   Classification of anorectal abscess and fistula-in-ano

I. Low intermuscular abscess
   (i.e) Infralevator-transsphincteric
      1. Perineal space
      2. Superficial postanal space
      3. Superficial anterior anal space
      4. Deep postanal space (horseshoe)
      5. Deep anterior anal space (horseshoe)
      6. Ischiorectal fossae
II. High intermuscular abscess
   (i.e.) Supralevator
      1. Retrorectal space
      2. Rectovesical space
      3. Pelvirectal space
III. Intermuscular abscess with combined supralevator and infralevator abscess
IV. Subcutaneous anal canal space
V. Submucosal rectal space

Source: reference 7.

cially in patients with AIDS. While at present there are no data available to determine what the percentages of these different anatomical classifications are in HIV-positive patients, it appears, at least in the author's experience, that complex fistulae as well as more extensive abscesses are more commonly seen in patients with impaired resistance.

Patients who are HIV-positive who present with ischiorectal abscesses must be considered true surgical emergencies. The risks of septicemia, Fournier's gangrene and other septic complications make immediate drainage imperative. However, one's aggressive approach must be tempered with a conservatism with regard to the extent of the open wounds simply because of the likelihood of poor healing in the operative site. As a result,

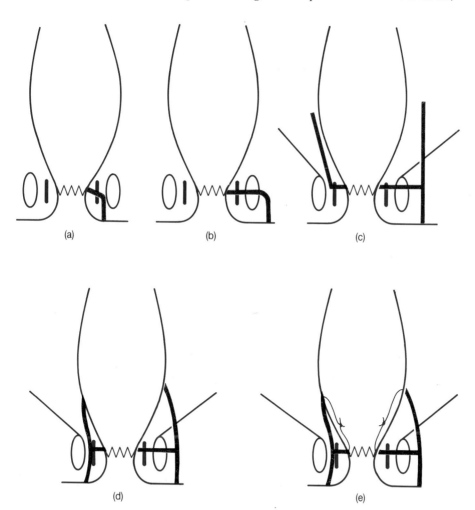

Figure 9.2 Fistulae-in-ano. (A) Intrasphincteric. (B) Transsphincteric. (C) Suprasphincteric. (D) Extrasphinteric. (E) shows the placement of setons in extrasphincteric fistulae-in-ano.

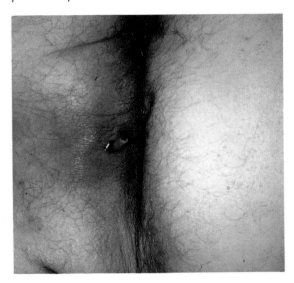

Figure 9.3   Simple catheter drainage of ischiorectal abscess.

simple catheter drainage—such as with 10Fr mushroom catheter—is sufficient for controling most simple abscesses (Fig. 9.3). For a more complex or phlegmonous process the ischiorectal space may be drained with multiple looped penrose drains (Figs 9.4A and 9.4B). Since the drains are sutured to themselves and lie flat, sitting is not uncomfortable. In this way the infectious process may be resolved (Fig. 9.5). A supralevator abscess can be drained by inserting a 12Fr Pezzer catheter through the levator ani musculature and bringing it out through the perianal skin (as seen in Fig. 9.3). Extrasphincteric tracts should be drained by heavy silk setons tied loosely (Figs 9.2E and 9.6). If the internal opening of the process is easily identified, the proximal 1 cm of the tract can be unroofed at the time of drainage, thus obviating the need for a separate fistulotomy at a later date (Fig. 9.7). These methods usually result in control of the infectious process. Broad-spectrum antibiotics should be included in the regimen. The drains are left in place until the entire indurated process has resolved, usually within two to three weeks. The drains are easily removed in an outpatient setting.

With regard to organisms cultured, no specific pattern has been seen in HIV-positive patients to date. A mixed population of aerobic and anaerobic bacteria is seen, at least in the author's experience. Commonly *B. fragilis*, *Pseudomonas*, *Klebsiella* and *E. coli* are seen. While cytomegalovirus (CMV) and *Mycobacterium avium intracellulare* (MAI) can be identified, these may represent contaminants from the GI tract rather than causative organisms. Both CMV and MAI frequently cause diarrhea and ulcerations in immunocompromised patients [10], and while both have resulted in small and large bowel perforations, the author has yet to find either as the primary cause of an ischiorectal abscess.

Fistulae-in-ano with or without ischiorectal abscesses are frequently multiple and complex in immunocompromised patients (Fig. 9.8A). Again, one

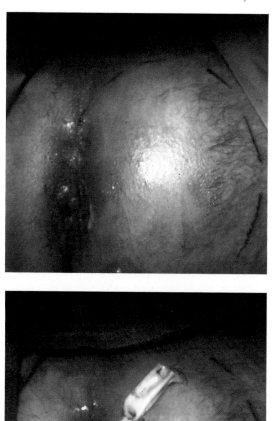

Figure 9.4 Large ischiorectal abscess in HIV patient. (A) The abscess and the limit of induration (dotted line). (B) Drainage of the abscess.

is committed to drainage of these chronically infected processes, but with the understanding that healing in the area is poor. One cannot simply unroof these tracts because the resulting operative defects may heal very slowly, if ever. Therefore, the proximal segment of the tract, if identified, is opened and the remaining tracts are curetted to remove as much granulation tissue as possible, irrigated, and narrow ribbon drains looped around the distal segments of the tracts (Fig. 9.8B). Depending on the level of the

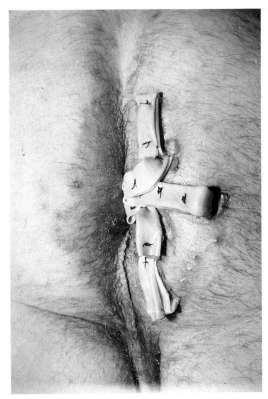

Figure 9.5 The infectious process resolved, and awaiting the removal of drains.

patients' resistance, these tracts will often heal when treated in this manner. The patient shown had nine separate fistulae, all of which were drained with eventual complete healing. (Note the perianal Kaposi sarcoma in the healed operative site—Fig. 9.8C.)

In a patient with an extrasphincteric fistula, unroofing of the segment above the puborectalis would result in incontinence which, in the immunocompromised state, would almost certainly be permanent and uncorrectable. Therefore any extension of the process in the vicinity of the sling cannot be cut. In these patients, as in those with extrasphincteric abscesses, the author has had success in placing heavy silk setons through both the internal opening and the extrasphincteric opening and loosely tying the sutures to themselves. These are not designed to cut through, since at best a large defect would be created that would probably never heal, and at worst, incontinence would result. However, by leaving these sutures tied loosely in place, drainage of any material that may accumulate is facilitated which prevents formation of recurrent abscesses. In addition, there is no discomfort since the patient is not even aware that the setons are in place. The author has had to use this technique twice in fourteen years in non-immunocompromised patients, both having Crohn's disease. For comparison purposes, in the last few months alone, this technique has had to be utilized three times in patients with AIDS. Not surprisingly, it appears that high fistulae are more prevalent in immunocompromised patients.

Wounds heal very slowly in this area in this patient population. The treatment of abscesses and fistulae has to be directed with this in mind. Wexner *et al.* [11] reported only a 12% incidence of healing in AIDS patients with anorectal problems. The poor results of aggressive management in their patients was reflected in a postoperative complication and mortality rate of 88% as opposed to less than a 5% incidence of complications following anorectal surgery in otherwise healthy individuals; 43% of their patients died within six months of treatment. These dismal results may reflect a specific patient population. The author has seen 22 HIV-positive patients with fistulae-in-ano with or without ischiorectal abscesses during the past two years. One patient died 19 days following emergency fistulotomy and drainage of abscess of advanced AIDS, a second died four months after undergoing fistulotomy and drainage of abscess. The other 20 have all done relatively well with symptomatic improvement in all cases and significant healing in 10. One patient was lost to long-term follow-up. Savari et al. [12] have, however, reported, over 90% healing of fistulae in HIV-positive patients in a recently published series.

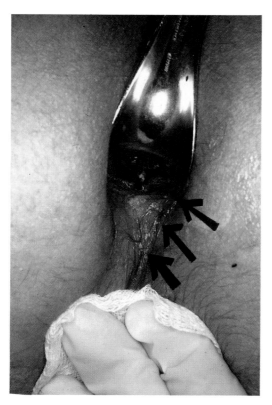

Figure 9.6 Use of a seton (arrows) for extrasphincteric fistula-in-ano (see Fig. 9.2E).

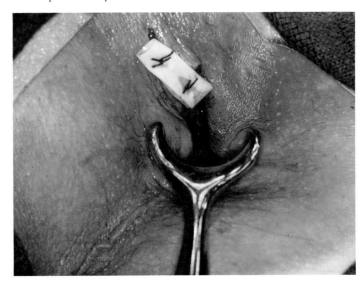

Figure 9.7   Single fistulous tract drained with primary segment unroofed.

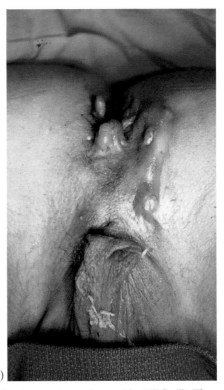

(a)

Figure 9.8   (A) Fistulae-in-ano in patient with AIDS. (B) The patient with drains inserted. (C) The healed fistulae (note the Kaposi sarcoma).

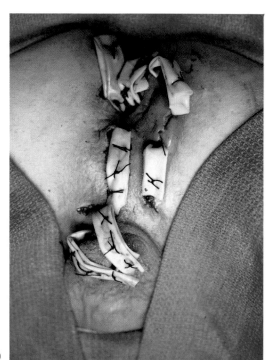

(b)

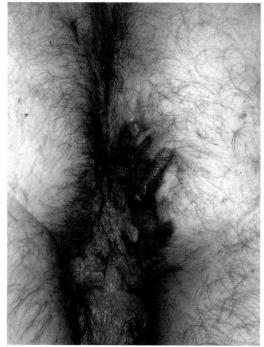

(c)

Conclusions

By the time it will have run its course, the human immunodeficiency virus will represent one of the great plagues of the twentieth century. Patients with AIDS deserve to be treated as humanely and compassionately as any other patients. The special problems in dealing with this patient population both from the standpoint of patients and concerned health-care workers make it mandatory that precautions be taken to protect everyone concerned. Patients with anal and perianal infections require expeditious care with regard to managing the infections combined with surgical conservatism since wounds in these patients heal poorly. A comprehensive study of the surgical management of HIV-positive patients with regard to predictability of healing based on readily comparable parameters has yet to be written. It is to be hoped that data in this regard will soon become available so as to improve the care of these unfortunate people and in some part lessen the terrible tragedy of AIDS.

References

1. Kaposi's sarcoma and pneumocystis pneumonia among homosexual men— New York City and California. *MMWR* 1981; **30**:305–8.
2. Weber DJ, Redfield RR, Leman SM. Acquired immunodeficiency syndrome: epidemiology and significance for the obstetrician and gynecologist. *Am J Obs Gyn* 1986; **155**:235–40.
3. Meyer AA. Surgical management of AIDS and HIV infected patients. *Adv Surg* 1989; **22**:57–73.
4. CDC: Recommendations for prevention of HIV transmission in health care settings. *MMWR* 1987; 35–185.
5. Meyer AA. AIDS: the disease and its relevance to surgeons. *Bull Am Coll Surg* 1986; **71**:11–17.
6. Corman ML. *Colon and Rectal Surgery.* Philadelphia: Lippencott, 1984: 104.
7. Hanley PH. Anorectal abscess fistula. *Surg Clin NA* 1978; **58**:487–503.
8. Parks AG, Gordon PH, Hardcastle JD. A classification of fistulae-in-ano. *Br J Surg* 1976; **63**:1–12.
9. Jones I, Fazio V, Jagelman D. Use of transanal rectal advancement flap in the management of fistulas involving the anorectum. *Dis Colon Rectum* 1987; **30**:919–23.
10. Hyder JW, MacKeigan JM. Anorectal and colonic disease and the immuno-compromised host. *Dis Colon Rectum* 1988; **31**:971–6.
11. Wexner SD, Smithy WB, Milsom JW, Dailey TH. The surgical management of-anorectal diseases in AIDS and pre-AIDS patients. *Dis Colon Rectum* 1986; **29**:719–23.
12. Safari A, Gottesman L, Dailey TH. Anorectal surgery in the HIV-positive patient: update. *Dis. Colon Rectum* (1991); **34**:299–304.

10

Warts and dysplasia
JH Scholefield and JMA Northover

Anal warts are reported to be 5–10 times more common than genital warts in homosexual men [1,2]. There are few published data on the prevalence of HPV infection among HIV infected patients, but it appears that anogenital HPV infection is particularly common in this group [3]. In the context of HIV infection, anogenital papillomavirus infection presents three main problems: the lesions are usually large in number, they may recur rapidly, and they may be more susceptible to dysplastic change. In view of the increasing number of HIV patients it seems likely that anogenital HPV infection will represent an increasing clinical problem both in numbers of patients and extent of disease in years to come.

Biology of human papillomaviruses

Papillomaviruses are classified as genus Papillomavirus of the *Papovaviridae* family (all are DNA viruses) on the basis of their capsid structure and biochemical composition [4]. They are relatively small DNA viruses and have icosahedral capsids about 55 nm in diameter. The DNA in these viruses is circular double-stranded, about 8000 base pairs in length, and contained as a central core within the protein capsid. DNA sequencing of papillomaviruses has demonstrated that they are markedly different from SV40, polyoma and other members of the papovavirus group and in future it may be more appropriate to regard the papillomaviruses as a distinct and unique family [5].

Molecular cloning and DNA sequencing have shown that all papillomaviruses share a similar genetic plan. The genetic code is contained within large overlapping open reading frames (ORFs) which are presenting only one strand (the 'sense strand') of the DNA. In common with other viruses the ORFs involved in cell transformation and viral replication are termed 'early' (E), while those ORFs coding for capsid proteins are termed 'late' (L). Between the E and L ORFs is a non-coding region of around 1000 base pairs which contains the genetic code for the viral regulatory elements; this is referred to as the 'upstream regulatory region' (URR).

In benign condylomata the viral chromosome is episomal, i.e. it is separate from the host genome. By contrast, in virally associated carcinomas, the viral genome is almost always integrated into the host DNA.

Since cellular transformation appears to be a function of the early regions of the genome [6,7], research has centered around this area of the viral DNA and its controlling elements in the URR. The E1 ORF controls viral replication, and the E2 ORF codes for a transacting factor which modulates viral gene expression from early region promoters, particularly for the E6 ORF. The E6 and E7 ORFs appear to be responsible for cellular transformation.

Papillomaviruses were first shown to be potentially oncogenic in the cottontail rabbit (CRPV—cottontail rabbit papillomavirus) [8]. Using this animal model, dramatic progress in understanding the carcinogenic potential of papillomaviruses was made by Rous and Beard [9]. They reported squamous cell carcinomas arising from Shope papillomavirus-induced warts on domestic rabbits. The rate of malignant conversion was found to be dependent upon viral strain, host species, and individual host. The frequency and speed of malignant conversion could also be influenced by the application of chemical carcinogens to the warty lesions. A further key development was the discovery of bovine papillomaviruses which cause esophageal and bladder cancer in cattle who eat bracken fern [10]. Bovine papillomaviruses were the first to be demonstrated to transform cells *in vitro*. The best characterized transformation assay is that of BPV1 which was shown to transform mouse cells C127 and NIH3T3 [11]. This system allowed the genetic dissection of the viral genes involved in cellular transformation. This information has been helpful in the study of human papillomavirus gene functions [12]. HPV type 16 has subsequently been shown to be capable of transforming the same cell lines as BPV1. In these animal models there can be little doubt that this group of viruses has malignant potential.

There are three clinicopathologic groups of human papillomaviruses:

(1) Cutaneotropic viruses found in immunologically normal individuals. These viruses produce benign infections which by definition can never be carcinogenic (e.g. HPV types 1, 2, 6, 11).
(2) Cutaneotropic viruses found in immunocompromised individuals. These HPV types can act synergistically with sunlight (or ultraviolet light) to cause malignant transformation. This occurs in a condition known as epidermodysplasia verruciformis (HPV types 5, 8, 12, 38).
(3) Mucosotropic viruses infecting the genital, oral and respiratory skin (HPV types 16, 18, 31, 33). The malignant potential of this group was unrecognized until about ten years ago when it was realized that many HPV infections are subclinical.

At the present time it has proven impossible to isolate living papillomavirus or to grow papillomaviruses in tissue culture, probably because of the complex host–virus interaction which cannot currently be reproduced *in vitro*.

Papillomaviruses are dependent upon the environment produced by the terminal differentiation of keratinocytes to complete their life-cycle. Although basal epithelial cells contain viral DNA, infectious virions are only found in the cells of the more superficial epithelium [13]. It may therefore be postulated that at specific stages in the cycle of viral replication epidermal growth factors may be necessary for viral replication. These factors may only be available through sequential differentiation of the host cells. Infection with papillomaviruses seems to require access to basal cells of the epithelium, and therefore local trauma may be important in facilitating papillomavirus infection. Infection may also be facilitated in actively dividing cells [5]. Such an area of rapid cellular division occurs at the transformation zone of the cervix which is thought to be particularly susceptible to HPV infection [14]. The cervical transformation zone lies between columnar and squamous epithelium and has a common embryologic derivation with the anal transitional zone [15,16], which may also be a site of predilection for HPV infection.

The complex nature of the interaction between the cycle of replication and the differentiation of the host cell is believed to be responsible for the difficulties in growing papillomaviruses in cell culture [17]. Consequently, demonstrating an association between papillomaviruses and human cancer has proved difficult experimentally; instead, DNA recombinant technology has been invaluable in the demonstration of the viral etiology of genital cancer.

The first consistent association of a human papillomavirus type with epidermodysplasia verruciformis (a rare form of human cancer) was reported by Orth and Jablonska [18]. They demonstrated the presence of HPV type 5 in squamous cell carcinoma in patients with epidermodysplasia verruciformis (EV). EV is a rare hereditary condition resulting in a defect in cell-mediated immunity which manifests as disseminated warts; on light-exposed sites some of these warts may become malignant. It has been suggested that this condition demonstrates the oncogenic potential of papillomaviruses in man [19].

Progress in HPV research was greatly facilitated by the introduction of molecular cloning procedures which led to the demonstration of differences in the DNA sequences in biologically different HPV types using DNA hybridization under conditions of 'high stringency' [20]. (In DNA hybridization technology, stringency refers to the pH, temperature and salt concentrations of the hybridization reactions which in turn determine the degree of sequence mismatching and stability of the DNA hybrids so formed.) The identification of the first specific genital HPV type, type 6 [21], was followed rapidly by the identification of additional anogenital types 11 [22], 16 [23], 18 [24], 31 [25], 33 [26] and several others more recently. At present 22 distinct HPV genotypes have been demonstrated in infections of the anogenital tract. HPV types 6, 11 and 42 are commonly found in genital warts, but HPV types 16, 18 and 33 are found in around 10% of warts (usually flat lesions) and these types have most commonly been associated with dysplastic lesions and invasive carcinomas. The predilection of different types for specific areas of the body has been noted—types 1 and 2 for hands and feet, types 6, 11 and 16 for the anogenital area—but are not fully understood. However, it seems likely that this tropism is due to a specific interaction between viral and cellular gene expression. HPV type 16 appears to be by far the most prevalent HPV type associated with cervical carcinoma (being found in more than 50% of cases). Cervical, vulvar and penile intraepithelial neoplasias (CIN, VIN, PIN) are considered to represent typical precursor lesions of cancers at these respective sites. Dysplastic change in association with HPV infection was first recognized on the cervix

[27]. Subsequently a grading system was developed, based on the number of thirds of the epithelial thickness which appear dysplastic on histologic section [28]. This grading has been adapted throughout the genital epithelium and has also been applied to the anus [29]. Colposcopic indices of dysplastic change have also been described [30]; though they serve as a useful guide, histology remains the definitive investigation. Recognition of those dysplastic lesions which have malignant potential from the vast majority of mild dysplasias which in the cervix do not appear to progress is a major difficulty in cervical screening. Currently little is known of the natural history of anal dysplastic lesions—studies are urgently required.

Little is known about the predilection of different HPV types for particular hosts. Studies of HPV infections in renal transplant recipients have shown that this group of immunosuppressed patients may be more susceptible to infection with the oncogenic HPV types (16 and 18) than immunologically normal hosts [31,32]. However, a study of the HPV types in anogenital lesions from 13 HIV infected patients has shown HPV types 6 and 11 to be the most prevalent types, while HPV type 16 DNA was not found in any of the 13 patients [33].

Epidemiology of papillomavirus infection

Very little is known about the epidemiology of papillomavirus infections in general. This is especially true for anal and genital papillomavirus infections which have for many years been surrounded by social and moral taboos.

The first description of warts was by Celsus in 25 AD. In the following five centuries, Greek and Roman physicians noted the sexual transmission of genital warts. Little was added to these observations for the next fifteen hundred years. Syphilis was a more serious problem for centuries and genital warts were not differentiated from condylomata lata, and therefore were regarded as a manifestation of syphilis. In 1793, Bell recognized that genital warts were unrelated to syphilis but thought they were a manifestation of gonorrhea [34]. This view persisted until the late nineteenth century when it was pointed out that many patients with warts gave no history of the other features of gonorrhea [35]. Following the clarification of the origin of gonorrhea through isolation of the gonococcus in 1879, irritants such as dirt, smegma or genital discharge were held responsible for causing warty epithelial proliferations on the genitalia. In 1893, Gemy described histologic similarities between skin warts and genital warts leading to the supposition that they shared a common origin [34].

In the nineteenth century anal warts were reported to be almost exclusively a disease of women already suffering from vulval warts. The suggestion of the association with anal intercourse arose in the late nineteenth century and subsequently in the early part of this century [36,37]. However, this was by no means a consensus view; Chester and Schwimmer [38] reported four cases in which there was 'no question of sodomy'. This controversy persists today with little objective evidence for either viewpoint. Apart from the taboos which for many years have surrounded sexually transmissible infections, understanding of papillomaviruses has also been hampered by difficulties in isolating the 'wart' virus, by the lack of a system of *in vitro* culture and by the variable incubation period of 1–20 months [39].

The viral origin of genital warts was first postulated by Cuiffo [40] who produced warts on his own hands by injecting a filtered extract of a genital wart. The sexually transmissible nature of genital condylomata was affirmed by Barrett *et al.* [41], who studied American servicemen returning from the Korean war, having acquired genital warts following intercourse with Korean women. Their wives developed genital condylomata following resumption of sexual activity. Sexual transmission of genital warts was confirmed by Oriel [1], who found a high incidence in the sexual contacts of patients with genital warts. He concluded that 'though anal coitus and anal warts are often associated, there may be other possible explanations for the occurrence of these warts'. This has recently received further support from Goorney [42] who reported that anal condylomata were common in hetero-sexual men. Goorney *et al.* demonstrated that 18 out of 60 heterosexual men (30%) with penile condylomata also had anal condylomata. In four of these cases the anal condylomata were above the level of the dentate line. They concluded that anal condylomata do not necessarily point to homosexual activity.

However, it has been noted that anal warts appear to be more common than penile warts among homosexual men [1,43]; this might suggest that the anus is a site of predilection for genital papillomaviruses. More recently Oriel has suggested that genital papillomaviruses may be a normal commen-sal in the anal canals of a proportion of the population and that condylomata may result from minor trauma in these susceptible individuals [44].

In the last 15 years there have been advances in the clinical, pathological and biochemical fields which have fundamentally changed our understand-ing of papillomaviruses and the conditions in which they are implicated. The first of these advances was the advent of the electron microscope in the 1940s. This enabled identification of details of papillomavirus structure; but more importantly the observation of virus particles in tissue provided further evidence for the viral origin of warts [45]. Viral particles were subsequently detected in genital warts by Dunn and Ogilvie in 1968 [46].

The histologic and cytologic description of the koilocyte (balloon cell), with its perinuclear vacuolation and nuclear hyperchromasia, and the arrival of molecular biological techniques have provided a fresh impetus to investigate the epidemiology of these viruses. DNA hybridization provides a sensitive and specific method for identification of papillomaviruses as well as a means of classifying the viral types.

Introduction of the operating microscope for the detection of subclinical papillomavirus infections and related dysplasias has led to an appreciation of the frequency of asymptomatic lesions [47].

Common plantar warts are usually caused by HPV type 1, and hand warts by HPV type 2. These viruses can be seen in desquamated epithelial cells using the electron microscope. Such cells are a major component in house-hold dust, and are thought to cause infection by entry through a small break in the epithelial surface. The infective potential of those types of human papillomavirus which infect the genital skin appears to be much lower than that of HPV types 1 and 2. The life-cycle of the papillomavirus is unlike that of any other virus. In man, papillomavirus infection is limited to the epidermis. In the normal epidermis only the basal cells divide; it seems likely, therefore, that the papillomavirus must infect these cells in order to multiply and infect other cells. It is postulated that the viral capsid proteins may recognize a cell surface receptor on basal cells. After entering, the virus probably undergoes limited replication, leading to a few copies of the virus in each infected cell. Thereafter there is probably synchronous viral replication and cellular division which allows the virus to maintain a foothold in all the daughter cells. Keratinocytes in the more superficial layers of the epidermis do not normally divide but differentiate progressively as the cells move outward in the epithelium. As the keratinocytes of the suprabasal layer ascend and undergo terminal differentiation, a new pattern of viral gene expression allows for a very high level of viral DNA replication and capsid production and the virus particles are assembled at this stage. Papillomaviruses cause hyperplasia in the intermediate layers (acanthosis).

Lorincz [25] demonstrated that individual HPV types which infect the cervix have varying degrees of oncogenic association. HPV types 6 and 11 were found to have little oncogenic potential compared with HPV types 16 and 18. The evidence of an etiological association between cervical cancer and HPV type 16 is increasingly compelling. Despite this association, HPV infection is probably only one of a number of events that occur in the pathogenesis of these tumors. In the last few years molecular virological evidence has suggested that anal squamous cell carcinoma may also be associated with HPV type 16 infection [48]. A further parallel between anal and cervical cancer has been demonstrated by reports of premalignant lesions in the anal canal which can be identified endoscopically; these lesions also contain HPV DNA [49,50]. Though there appears to be a spectrum of anal lesions, from the benign infection through grades of mild dysplasia (AIN I) to carcinoma-in-situ (AIN III), the natural history of these lesions and the proportion which progress to invasive carcinoma is unknown. Studies of the natural history of cervical intraepithelial neoplasia have shown that progression of CIN III to invasive carcinoma may occur in up to 25% of cases over a 20-year follow-up period [51]. Studies of the natural history of anal dysplastic lesions are awaited.

Syrjanen [52] reported that anal condylomata are most commonly associated with HPV types 6 and 11 DNA, but that types 16 and 18 are also found. The finding that some anal cancers contain integrated HPV type 16 DNA [48] demonstrates a parallel between anal and cervical squamous cell carcinomas. Since these particular papillomavirus types are known to be sexually transmissible, it follows that the development of anal squamous cell carcinoma is preceded by infection with a potentially oncogenic HPV type such as HPV 16. From existing epidemiologic evidence it seems that genital HPV infection requires intimate contact, possibly on more than one occasion. Once the genital skin is infected the localization of the infection is poorly understood. Experiments by Ferenczy [53] have shown that HPV DNA can be detected in small amounts in normal skin up to 2 cm away from macroscopic lesions (microscopic examination of the 'normal skin' was not

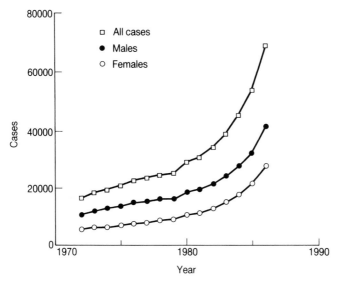

Figure 10.1   The increasing incidence of genital condylomata from 1970 to 1986 [54].

performed) and suggests that these subclinical lesions may subsequently become overt condylomata.

There has been an alarming increase in the prevalence of genital HPV infections, both in the UK (Fig. 10.1) [54] and in the USA [55]. These trends, together with increasing evidence for the oncogenic potential of certain HPV types, makes understanding the epidemiology of these infections essential. Information on the possible interactions between HIV infection and possible HPV infection is sparse. However, it is becoming apparent that HIV infection may predispose the individual to unusual HPV infections [56]. It remains to be seen what the natural history of such infections may be.

The incidence of invasive anal cancer is said to be increasing in HIV-positive men [57], but the evidence for this statement is limited. In the most recent epidemiological study of anal cancer, Daling [58] reported a case–control study in which the relative risk of anal cancer was increased 33-fold in men with a history of anal intercourse compared with a control group with colon cancer; no information on HIV infection was reported. (HPV 16 DNA was identified in approximately 30% of the anal cancers in this study using *in situ* hybridization; see Beckmann [59].) Several studies have described immunosuppressed patients as being at increased risk of cervical intraepithelial neoplasia [60,61]; similar findings have been recorded for the anal epithelium in HIV-positive men [62,50]. Further studies are awaited with interest.

Diagnosis of anogenital HPV infections

Papillomavirus infections are often asymptomatic; the most common symptom is one of cosmetic deformity. However, some patients complain of pruritus and occasional bleeding. Pruritus is probably due to difficulty in keeping the affected skin clean particularly in the perianal area; bleeding usually results from minor trauma arising from defecation. Large lesions may become colonized by bacteria and produce foul-smelling discharge.

Clinically apparent papillomavirus infections may be condylomatous, papular or flat keratotic plaques. Frequently several of these types exist in the same individual.

(1) Classic *condylomata acuminata* predominate in moist areas such as the anal canal epithelium, vulva and prepuce. Each lesion comprises a number of villous projections. Colour may vary from red through pink to gray depending on the vascularity of the papillae.
(2) More rounded *papular warts* predominate in drier areas of skin such as the shaft of the penis or the hair-bearing perianal skin. These lesions tend to be more heavily keratinized and therefore rather paler than the surrounding skin.
(3) *Flat keratotic plaques* are sessile lesions which may be easily overlooked by the clinician. Their contour is usually minimally raised above the surrounding epithelium.

The recognition of *subclinical papillomavirus infection* is a relatively recent phenomenon; the prevalence of these lesions continues to increase as more clinicians adopt the techniques of examination of the anal and genital epithelia under magnification after soaking in acetic acid [30]. Subclinical papillomavirus lesions are by definition those which can only be seen with the aid of special diagnostic techniques, i.e. the application of acetic acid and viewing under magnification. There is a technical difference between examining the cervix and examining the genital and perianal epithelium in that the latter areas often require soaking in acetic acid for 3–5 minutes before HPV-related lesions become apparent. This may account for under-reporting of subclinical lesions in many studies. The appearances of the subclinical lesion may be merely an aceto-whitened area of epithelium but subclinical intraepithelial neoplasia occurs. Distinction between a truly benign aceto-white lesion and mild intraepithelial neoplasia is ultimately made by histologic examination, but intraepithelial neoplasia may also be assessed using examination with acetic acid and magnification using the criteria described by Reid *et al.* [30]. These features are based on the color, vascular pattern, surface configuration and topographical anatomy of the lesions.

Management of anogenital HPV infections

In view of the description of HPV-associated premalignant lesions in the anal canal and perianal skin, and the prospect that HIV infected individuals are at increased risk of dysplastic change in condylomatous lesions, the authors believe that the clinician should have a low threshold of suspicion and that biopsy should be undertaken for any endoscopically abnormal lesion or alternatively for any condylomatous lesion which has an atypical appearance. The authors have undertaken several hundred biopsies of potentially dysplastic lesions in the anal canal and perianal area, under local anesthetic (2% lignocaine with 1:300 000 adrenalin) using a modified 5 mm Ajax rangeur without undue discomfort to the patient and without sequelae. In a study of patients with anal HPV infection, 29% of patients were found to have dysplastic change; 7% were AIN III [50]. Local excision or laser therapy of premalignant lesions are the treatments of choice.

In immunosuppressed individuals HPV infection and HPV-associated malignancies seem to be more prevalent than in the population at large. Furthermore, widespread infection with atypical HPV types has been reported in such patients [63]. Anal condylomata are 5–10 times more common than genital condylomata in homosexual men [2]. In HIV-antibody-positive men, anal and genital HPV infections are often extensive [64] and even more difficult to eradicate than in the immunologically normal individual [65]. In view of the association between HPV infection and HIV in homosexual men, the San Francisco Mens' Health Study has examined the association between HIV seropositivity and HPV infection to determine whether HPV infection may predispose to seroconversion. They found that HPV infection does not predispose to seroconversion but may be a marker of patients at risk of HIV seroconversion [3].

In asymptomatic HIV-antibody-positive (CDC stage 2) individuals, attempts to eradicate condylomata are not likely to succeed, but debulking extensive condylomata will improve the patient's symptoms and may lessen the risk of subsequent malignancy. Once debulked the lesions may be kept under control by regular outpatient therapy using either excision, diathermy or cryotherapy. Podophyllin should probably not be used in these patients as it is generally ineffective, can have severe systemic effects and may induce dysplastic changes in condylomata [66].

In symptomatic HIV-positive (CDC stage 3) individuals, conservative treatment of condylomata is advised because, as in other forms of perianal disease, postoperative healing is impaired [57,67,68]. However, biopsy and histologic examination of a suspicious lesion are indicated as dysplastic change is commonly seen in patients in this group with condylomata [69,62]. The natural history of these dysplasias has not been fully established, but centers dealing with large homosexual populations report an increase in the incidence of both carcinoma-in-situ and invasive anal squamous cell carcinoma [69,70].

In patients with AIDS (CDC stage 4), anal condylomata are often extensive and recurrence is likely, soon after excision. Furthermore, excision of condylomata in this group is frequently complicated by delayed healing [69,68]. Therefore, in patients with AIDS the only reasonable procedure for condylomata is biopsy of a lesion suspected of being a carcinoma. Many of these biopsies will show dysplastic changes of varying severity, even carcinoma-in-situ; but in view of the poor healing following surgery no further procedures should be undertaken. Invasive carcinoma is probably best managed by radiotherapy.

References

1. Oriel JD. Anal warts and anal coitus. *Br J Vener Dis* 1971; **47**:373–6.
2. Judson FN, Penley KA, Robinson ME, Smith JK. Comparative prevalence rates of sexually transmitted diseases in heterosexual and homosexual men. *Am J Epidemiol* 1980; **112**:836–43.
3. Kent C, Samuel M, Winkelstein J. The role of anal/genital warts in HIV infection. *JAMA* 1987; **258**:3385–6.
4. Matthews REF. Classification and nomenclature of viruses. *Intervirology* 1982; **17**:1–199.
5. Broker TR, Botchan M. Papillomaviruses: retrospectives and prospectives. In Botchan M, Grodzicker T, Sharp PA (eds), *DNA Tumor Viruses: Control of Gene Expression and Replication*. Cold Spring Harbor Laboratory, New York: 1986; **4**:17–36.
6. Giri I, Danos O. Papillomavirus genomes: from sequence data to biological properties. *TIG* 1986; Sept: 227–32.
7. Matlashewski G, Schneider J, Banks, L, Jones M, Murray A, Crawford LV. Human papillomavirus type 16 DNA cooperates with activated ras in transforming primary cells. *EMBO J* 1987; **6**:1741–6.
8. Shope RE, Weston Hurst E. Infectious papillomatosis of rabbits; with a note on the histopathology. *J Exp Med* 1933: **58**:607–24.
9. Rousb P, Beard JW. The progression to carcinoma of virus induced rabbit papillomas (Shope). *J Exp Med* 1935; **62**:523–45.
10. Pfister H. Biology and biochemistry of papillomaviruses. *Rev Physiol Biochem Pharmacol* 1984; **99**:111–81.
11. Dvoretzky I, Sheober R, Chattopahyay SK, Lowy DR. A quantitative *in vitro* assay for bovine papillomavirus. *Virology* 1980; **130**:369–75.
12. Howley PM, Schlegel R. The human papillomaviruses: an overview. *Am J Med* 1988; **85**:155–8.
13. Orth G, Favre M, Croissant O. Characterization of a new type of human papillomavirus that causes skin warts. *J Virol* 1977; **24**:108–20.
14. Koss LG. Cytologic and histologic manifestations of human papillomavirus infection of the female genital tract and their clinical significance. *Cancer* 1987; **60**:1942–50.
15. Tench EM. Development of the anus in the human embryo. *Am J Anat* 1936; **59**:333–45.
16. Grinvalsky HT, Helwig EB. Carcinoma of the anorectal junction. *Cancer* 1956; **9**:480–8.
17. Taichman LB, Reilly SS, LaPorta RF. The role of keratinocyte differentiation in the expression of epitheliotropic viruses. *J Invest Dermatol* 1983; **81**:137s–140s.
18. Orth G, Jablonska S, Favre M, Croissant O, Jarzabek-Chorzelska M, Rzesa G. Characterization of two types of human papillomaviruses in lesions of epidermodysplasia verruciformis. *Proc Natl Acad Sci USA* 1978; **75**:1537–41.
19. Orth G. Epidermodysplasia verruciformis: a model for understanding the oncogenicity of human papillomaviruses. *Ciba Foundation Symposium* 1986; **120**:157–74.
20. Heilmann CA, Law M-F, Israel MA, Howley PM. Cloning of human papillomavirus DNAs and analysis of homologous polynucleotide sequences. 1980; **36**:395–407.
21. Gissmann L, zur Hausen. H. Partial characterization of viral DNA from human genital warts (condylomata acuminata). *Int J Cancer* 1980; **25**:605–609.
22. Gissmann L, Diehl V, Schultz-Coulon H-J, zur Hausen H. Molecular cloning

and characterization of human papilloma virus DNA derived from a laryngeal papilloma. *J Virol* 1982; **44**:393–400.

23. Durst M, Gissman L, Ikenberg H, zur Hausen H. Papillomavirus DNA from a cervical carcinoma and its prevalence in cancer biopsy samples from different geographical regions. *Proc Natl Acad Sci USA* 1983; **80**:3812–15.

24. Boshart M, Gissmann L, Ikenberg H, Kleinheuinz A, Scheurlen W, zur Hausen H. A new type of papillomavirus DNA, its presence in genital cancer biopsies and in cell lines derived from cervical cancer. *EMBO J* 1984; **3**:1151–7.

25. Lorincz A, Temple GF, Kurman RJ. Oncogenic association of specific human papillomavirus types and cervical neoplasia. *JNCI* 1987; **79**:671–7.

26. Beaudenon S, Kremsdorf D, Obalek S, Jablonska S, *et al*. Plurality of genital human papillomaviruses: characterization of two new types with distinct biological properties. *Virology* 1987; **161**:374–84.

27. Meisels A, Fortin R. Condylomatous lesions of the cervix and vagina. I. Cytologic patterns. *Acta Cytologica* 1976; **20**:505–509.

28. Richart RM. Cervical intraepithelial neoplasia. *Path Ann* 1973; **8**:301–328.

29. Fenger C. The anal transitional zone. *Acta Path Microbiol Scand Sect A* 1979; **87**:379–386.

30. Reid R, Stanhope CR, Angronov SJ. Genital warts and cervical cancer. IV: A colposcopic index for differetiating subclinical papillomavirus infection from cervical intraepithelial neoplasia. *Am J Obstet* Gynecol 1984; **149**:815–19.

31. Rudlinger R, Smith IW, Bunney MH, *et al*. Human papillomavirus infections in a group of renal transplant patients. *Br J Dermatol* 1986; **115**:681–92.

32. Lutzner MA, Orth G, Dutronquay G. Detection of human papillomavirus type 5 DNA in skin cancer of an immunosuppressed renal allograft recipient. *Lancet* 1983, **ii**:422.

33. Rudlinger R, Grob R, Buchmann P, Christen D, Steiner R. Anogenital warts of the condyloma acuminatum type in HIV positive patients. *Dermatologica* 1988; **176**:277–81.

34. Oriel JD. Natural history of genital warts. *Br J Vener Dis* 1971; **47**:1–13.

35. Ravogli A. Genital warts and gonorrhoea. *JAMA* 1916; **67**:109–113.

36. Parnell RJG. Observations upon the venereal lesions of the rectum and anus. *J Roy Nav Med Serv* 1929; **15**:77–84.

37. Drueck CJ. Papilloma about the anal region. *Urol Cutan Rev* 1941; **45**:581–3.

38. Chester BJ, Schwimmer B. Perianal veruca acuminata with mucosal lesions. *Arch Derm* 1955; **71**:149.

39. Laurent R, Kienzler JL. Epidemiology of HPV infections. *Clin Dermatol* 1985; **43**:64–70.

40. Cuiffo G. Innesto positivo con filtradi di verrucae vulgare. *Giorno Ital Mal Venereol* 1907; **48**:12–17.

41. Barrett TJ, Silba, JD, McGinley J. Genital warts—a venereal disease. *JAMA* 1954; **154**:333–5.

42. Goorney BD, Waugh MA, Clarke J. Anal warts in heterosexual men. *Genitourin Med* 1987; **63**:216.

43. Carr G, William DC. Anal warts in a population of gay men in New York City. *Sex Trans Dis* 1977; **4**:56–7.

44. Oriel JD. Condylomata acuminata as a sexually transmitted disease. *Dermatol Clin* 1983; **1**:93–102.

45. Strauss MJ, Shaw EW, Bunting H, Melnick JK. 'Crystalline' virus-like particles from ski papillomas characterised by intra-nuclear inclusion bodies. *Proc Soc Exp Biol Med* 1949; **72**:46–51.

46. Dunn AEG, Ogilvie MM. Intranuclear virus particles in human genital wart tissue: observations on the ultrastructure of the epidermal layer. *J Ultrastructure Res* 1968; **22**:282–95.

47. Reid R, Stanhope CR, Herschmann BR. Genital warts and cervical cancer I. *Cancer* 1982; **50**:377–87.
48. Palmer JG, Scholefield JH, Coates PJ, Shepherd NA, Jass JR, Crawford LV, Northover JMA. Anal squamous cell carcinoma and human papillomaviruses. *Dis Col Rectum* 1989; **32**:1016–22.
49. McCance DJ, Clarkson PK, Dyson JL, Walker PG, Singer A. Human papillomavirus types 6 and 16 in multifocal intraepithelial neoplasias of the female lower genital tract. *Br J Obstet Gynaecol* 1985; **92**:1093–100.
50. Scholefield JH, Sonnex C, Talbot IC, *et al*. Anal and cervical intra-epithelial neoplasia: possible parallels. *Lancet* 1989; **ii**:765–9.
51. McIndoe WA, McLean MR, Jones RW, Mullins PR. The invasive potential of carcinoma-in-situ of the cervix. *Obst Gynaecol* 1984; **64**:451–8.
52. Syrjanen K, Syrjanen S, von Krogh G. Anal condylomas in homosexual/bisexual and heterosexual males. II: Histopathological and virological assessment. *VIIth Int Papillomavirus Workshop* 1988: 127.
53. Ferenczy A, Mitao M, Naga N, Silverstein SJ. Latent papillomavirus and recurring genital warts. *New Engl J Med* 1985; **313**:784–8.
54. Communicable Disease Surveillance Centre. Sexually transmitted disease surveillance in Britain 1984. *Br Med J* 1986; **296**:942–3.
55. Becker TM. Genital warts–a sexually transmitted disease (STD) epidemic?. *Colp Gynae Laser Surg* 1984; **1**:193–7.
56. Greenspan D, de Villiers EM, Greenspan, JS, de Souza YG, zur Hausen H. Unusual HPV types in oral warts in association with HIV infection. *J Oral Pathol* 1988; **17**:482–7.
57. Wexner SD, Smithy WB, Milsom JW, Dailey TH. The surgical management of anorectal disease in AIDS and the pre-AIDS patients. *Dis Colon Rectum* 1986; **29**:719–23.
58. Daling JR, Weiss NS, Hislop PHTG, Maden C, Coates RJ, Sherman KJ, Ashley RL, Beagrie M, Ryan JA, Corey L. Sexual practices, sexually transmitted diseases, and the incidence of anal cancer. *New Engl J Med* 1987; **317**:973–7.
59. Beckmann AM, Daling JR, Sherman KJ, *et al*. Human papillomavirus infection and anal cancer. *Int J Cancer* 1989; **3**(4):1042–9.
60. Maclean AB, Lynn KL, Bailey, *et al*. Colposcopic assessment of lower genital tract in female transplant recipients. *Clin Nephrol* 1986; **26**:45–57.
61. Cordinger JW, Sharp F, Briggs JD. Cervical intraepithelial neoplasia in immunosuppressed women after renal transplantation. *Scott Med J* 1980; **25**:275–77.
62. Frazer IH, Crapper RM, Medley G, Brown TC, Makay IR. Association between anorectal dysplasia, human papillomavirus and HIV infection in homosexual men. *Lancet* 1986; **ii**:657–70.
63. Milburn PB, Brandsma JL, Goldman CI, Teplitz ED, Heilman EI. Disseminated warts in a patient with acquired immunodeficiency syndrome. *J Am Acad Dermatol* 1989; **19**:401–5.
64. Schneider V, Kay S, Lee HM. Immunosuppression as a high risk factor in the development of condyloma acuminatum and squamous neoplasia of the cervix. *Acta Cytologica* 1983; **27**:220–5.
65. McMillan A, Bishop PE. Clinical course of anogenital warts in men infected with human immunodeficiency virus. *Genitourin Med* 1989; **65**:225–8.
66. Wade TR, Ackerman AB. The effects of resin of podophyllin on condyloma accuminatum. *Am J Dermatopathol* 1984; **6**(2):109–22.
67. Hyder JW, MacKeigan JM. Anorectal and colonic disease in the immuno-compromised host. *Dis Col Rectum* 1988; **31**:971–6.
68. Carr ND, Mersey D, Slack WW. Non-condylomatous perianal disease in homosexual men. *Br J Surg* 1989; **76**:1064–6.

69. Croxon T, Chabon AB, Rorat E, Barash IM. Intra epithelial carcinoma of the anus in homosexual men. *Dis Col Rectum* 1984; **27**:325–30.
70. Wexner SD, Milsom JW, Dailey TH. The demographics of anal cancer are changing. *Dis Col Rectum* 1987; **30**(12):942–6.

11

Anorectal neoplasia
Craig E Metroka and Alvaro Vallejo

Introduction

The acquired immunodeficiency syndrome (AIDS) is a disorder which, in the USA, is seen predominantly in male homosexuals. It is characterized by life-threatening opportunistic infections, Kaposi's sarcoma, and is associated with a deficiency in cell-mediated immunity. AIDS is caused by a retrovirus that is lymphotropic for helper T cells (CD4+) and impairs the function of these cells, resulting in increased susceptibility to opportunistic infections [1,2]. Reversal of the immune dysfunction does not occur spontaneously in patients with AIDS, and the syndrome appears to be invariably fatal.

AIDS, as defined by the Centers for Desease Control (CDC), probably identifies a small segment of a larger population presenting with generalized lymphadenopathy, autoimmune disorders, Hodgkin's disease, and possibly for certain other malignancies, that should be included within a broader definition. The clinical outcome for all these patients depends on the severity of their immune dysfunction; exposure to, or reactivation of, common pathogens; genetic and other host factors; and the strain or rate of mutation of HIV. (See Table 11.1.)

Anorectal problems may occur in any HIV infected patient, but they are

Table 11.1 Neoplasms associated with HIV infection

Definite neoplasms associated with HIV infection
  Non-Hodgkin's lymphoma
  Kaposi's sarcoma
  Squamous-cell carcinoma

Other Neoplasms that may be associated with HIV infection
  Hodgkin's disease
  Cloacogenic carcinoma
  Condyloma acuminatum
  Malignant melanoma
  Hepatocellular carcinoma
  Adenocarcinoma of the lung, stomach, small bowel, colon, and rectum

particularly common among homosexual men. This review summarizes the rectal malignancies that can be seen in homosexual men with evidence of immune dysfunction and the possible treatments that are available to them.

Kaposi's sarcoma

Origin of Kaposi's sarcoma

Study of the biology and pathogenesis of Kaposi's sarcoma has been hampered by the inability to maintain long-term cultures of Kaposi's sarcoma cells. Gallo and associates have shown that spindle cells from Kaposi's sarcoma lesions can be grown in long-term culture by initiating and supporting their growth with conditioned media (CM) derived from activated human CD4+ cells infected with either HTLV-I, HTLV-II, or HIV-1 infected CD4+ cells [3–5]. Morphological and immunohistochemical studies indicated that the Kaposi's sarcoma cells were mesenchymal cell in origin and had features in common with endothelial and smooth muscle cells (Fig. 11.1) [4]. Using this cell culture system they showed that the Kaposi's sarcoma-derived cells produce biological activities which promote self-growth, growth of normal endothelial cells, fibroblasts and other cell types, new blood vessel formation, and chemotactic and chemoinvasive factors for Kaposi's sarcoma cells and normal cells [4,5]. An animal model was developed in which the induction of mouse lesions, closely resembling human Kaposi's sarcoma, were obtained by transplantation of human Kaposi's sarcoma cells in nude mice. Surprisingly, the tumors obtained were mouse in origin [6].

While there is a direct correlation between HIV-1 infection and the development of Kaposi's sarcoma in AIDS patients, the mechanism by

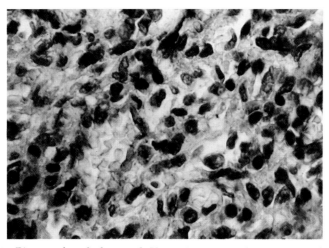

Figure 11.1   Biopsy of anal ulcer with Kaposi's sarcoma (microscopic) featuring spindle-shaped cells.

which HIV-1 induces these tumors is not yet understood. The ability of the AIDS-Kaposi's sarcoma cells to grow with CM derived from HIV-1 infected cells to induce Kaposi's sarcoma-like lesions in mice, and the high incidence of Kaposi's sarcoma in HIV-1 infected individuals, strongly suggests a link between Kaposi's sarcoma and HIV-1 infection. However, since HIV-1 sequences are not found in the DNA from Kaposi's sarcoma tissue or in cells isolated from the tumor [4], the role of HIV-1 in Kaposi's sarcoma is probably indirect and due to a paracrine effect exerted by the infected cells. In addition, Vogel *et al.* showed that the tat gene of HIV-1 introduced into the germ line of mice induced skin lesions resembling Kaposi's sarcoma [6]. Although the development of tumors is correlated with the expression of tat in the skin of the animals, the tumor cells do not express the tat gene, suggesting the presence of a paracrine mechanism of tumor induction. Consequently, it is possible that the Kaposi's sarcoma growth promoting activity present in CM from HIV-1 infected cells might be tat itself and the tat protein could be released by infected cells and might directly promote AIDS–Kaposi's sarcoma cell growth or indirectly by activating target cells to express growth promoting gene(s). These data support a model that *in vivo* factor(s) released by HIV-1 infected cells initiate and maintain cellular events that lead to the production of cytokines and the consequent cell growth and histologic changes characteristic of AIDS–Kaposi's sarcoma. Recently, another hypothesis raised the possibility that Kaposi's sarcoma was caused by another sexually transmitted disease (virus) based on the observation that Kaposi's sarcoma developed in individuals who were at risk for AIDS but were negative for antibody for HIV [7,8].

Clinical presentation and diagnosis

AIDS-related Kaposi's sarcoma is characterized by the sudden and often widespread occurrence of lesions at the onset of the disease, involving the skin, oral mucosa, lymph nodes and visceral organs. The mucocutaneous lesions are usually asymptomatic, may be single or multiple, and sometimes appear simultaneously or sequentially. New lesions may continue to appear throughout the course of the disease. However, no predictor has been found to determine which patients will develop Kaposi's sarcoma and the rate that the lesions will appear. No correlation has been observed with the number of CD4+ cells and the development of Kaposi's sarcoma (EC Metroka unpublished observations). As the lesions become more numerous, they tend to occur in a bilateral symmetrical distribution along the lines of skin cleavage. The lesions are often elongated, fusiform, or oval in shape. As these tumors evolve, the flat lesions become elevated, developing into papules or plaques (plaque stage). Eventually, the plaque stage lesions may enlarge, coalesce and become elevated nodules (nodular stage). Kaposi's sarcoma has rarely been reported in the central nervous system.

Although Kaposi's sarcoma is rarely a direct cause of death in HIV infected patients, the morbidity associated with more advanced disease can be significant. Bulky cutaneous lesions may become painful and, if large cutaneous surfaces are involved, may restrict movement. Lymphatic obstruction is common and may result in edema, most commonly involving the extremities or the face. Visceral spread of Kaposi's sarcoma is rarely symptomatic, particularly when it involves the gastrointestinal tract. However, rare cases of obstruction of gastrointestinal bleeding have been reported. Most gastrointestinal Kaposi's sarcoma lesions are discovered incidentally during endoscopic procedures. Endoscopic biopsy of Kaposi's sarcoma lesions is safe; no complications have been reported. The yield of endoscopic biopsy is relatively low. Overall the likelihood of a positive biopsy of a characteristic lesion is only about 25% [9]. The low yield is probably due to the submucosal location of the tumor, which makes it inaccessible to the standard biopsy instrument. A digital rectal examination is important in the evaluation of a patient who is HIV-positive since the presence of a nodule on rectal examination may be the first clue to the presence of Kaposi's sarcoma. Although visceral Kaposi's sarcoma lesions rarely cause symptoms, patients with gastrointestinal involvement by Kaposi's sarcoma have a poorer prognosis than those without visceral involvement [9]. Massive bleeding from GI tract lesions can rarely occur and requires prompt treatment.

In contrast, pulmonary Kaposi's sarcoma may cause cough, bronchospasm, and dyspnea. The constellation of signs and symptoms of cough, dyspnea, hemoptysis or the presence of blood-tinged sputum, with pulmonary infiltrates on chest x-ray and a negative gallium scan, is virtually diagnostic of pulmonary involvement with Kaposi's sarcoma. This is one of the few instances when Kaposi's sarcoma is life-threatening and aggressive chemotherapy is warranted.

Staging

Currently employed staging systems are based primarily on tumor bulk. Unfortunately, these systems have not proven useful because a majority of patients fall into advanced stages. In addition, tumor bulk may not be the most important predictor of survival and immunological parameters may prove more useful.

Based upon these known predictors of survival in AIDS-associated Kaposi's sarcoma, the Oncology Subcommittee of the NIAID sponsored AIDS Clinical Trials Group (ACTG) has proposed a new staging classification (Table 11.2) [10]. This system takes into account the extent of tumor, the status of the immune function as assessed by CD4+ cell count, and the severity of the systemic illness, including history of opportunistic infections and the presence of constitutional symptoms. It will require validation in future prospective clinical trials. If this staging classification proves useful, its use will facilitate trial design and analysis.

Current recommendations for treatment

Table 11.3 summarizes our recommendations for treatment of patients with Kaposi's sarcoma. Patients with minimal disease, unless cosmetically unsightly or painful, are generally not candidates for Kaposi's sarcoma-directed therapy. Those patients may benefit from zidovidine or other

Table 11.2   Recommended staging classification

	Good risk (0) (any of the following)	Poor risk (1) (any of the following)
Tumor (T)	Confined to skin and/or lymph nodes and/or minimal oral disease*	Tumor-associated edema or ulceration Extensive oral KS Gastrointestinal KS KS in other non-nodal viscera
Immune system (I)	CD4+ cells $\geqslant 200/mm^3$	CD4+ cells $\leqslant 200/mm^3$
Systemic illness (S)	No history of OI or thrush No 'B' symptoms† performance status $\geqslant 70$ (Karnofsky)	History of OI and/or thrush 'B' symptoms present Performance status $\leqslant 70$ Other HIV-related (e.g. neurological disease, lymphoma)

*Minimal oral disease is non-nodular KS confined to the palate
†'B' symptoms are unexplained fever, night sweats, >10% involuntary weight loss, or diarrhea persisting more than 2 weeks
Source: reference 10

experimental antiretrovirals or immunomodulators as they become available. Systemic therapy is recommended for patients with asymptomatic but progressive disease or for patients with widespread symptomatic or pulmonary disease.

Adriamycin-containing regimens should generally be reserved for patients with more advanced disease or patients with previously unsuccessful therapy. Vincristine with or without bleomycin may benefit those patients with neutropenia. Locally symptomatic disease can be palliated with

Table 11.3   Recommendations for treatment of Kaposi's sarcoma

Minimal disease	
Stable or slowly progressive	Observation only Investigational drugs—antivirals and immunomodulators Zidovudine
Rapidly progressive	Vinblastine ± bleomycin Vepesid Alpha interferon (in patients with >200 CD4+ cells/mm³)
Widespread, symptomatic	Adriamycin, bleomycin, and vincristine
Pulmonary Kaposi's sarcoma	Adriamycin, bleomycin, and vincristine
Locally symptomatic	Radiotherapy Laser (oral lesions)
Local cosmesis	Radiotherapy Intralesional vinblastine Cryotherapy
Neutropenic patients	Vincristine alternating with bleomycin

localized therapy, generally radiation. However, radiation should be used with caution for oral lesions and possibly rectal tumors. Large, bulky rectal tumors or other bulky disease involving the GI tract has been successfully treated at our institution with Nd:YAG laser photocoagulation [11]. Frequently, chemotherapy has to be used after the tumor has been reduced in size, to prevent recurrent disease. Local cosmetic problems may be successfully treated with intralesional velban or cryotherapy. However, the best cosmetic results are obtained when treatment is given when the lesions are small (<5 mm). Alpha-interferon as a single agent may be considered in those patients with more intact immune function (CD4+cells >200/mm^3). Alpha-interferon has no role in the management of patients with life-threatening visceral disease. The use of alpha-interferon and zidovudine or another antiviral together may also prove efficacious. However, widespread use of these agents in combination should await the results of large clinical trials currently in progress. The use of chemotherapy in combination with zidovudine should be used with caution because of the high risk of neutropenia. Our experience suggests that the only chemotherapeutic agent that can be safely used with zidovudine is bleomycin. In addition, all patients with fewer than 200 CD4+ cells/mm^3 should be placed on prophylaxis for pneumocystis using either Bactrim double-strength 1 tablet twice-daily, dapsone 25 mg four times daily, or aerosolized pentamidine 300 mg monthly. Prophylaxis for other opportunistic infections (i.e. toxoplasmosis, disseminated fungal infections, cytomegalovirus disease, and *Mycobacterium avium intracellulare*) is presently under investigation both through the ACTG and the Community Based Clinical Trials (CBCT).

Non-Hodgkin's lymphoma

Clinical presentation

The typical features of non-Hodgkin's lymphoma in HIV-positive individuals include young age at presentation, aggressive (high-grade) histologic types, the presentation at extranodal sites, and at advanced stage according to the Ann Arbor Staging System at the time of presentation [12]. As a result of involvement of multiple organ systems the manifestations of disease can be quite diverse. Local or systemic symptoms may predominate.

In the case of GI tract lymphoma, signs and symptoms can arise from primary GI tract involvement, or from direct extension of abdominal lymphadenopathy. Presenting complaints include GI bleeding, dysphagia, ulcer symptoms, bowel obstruction, obstipation, gingival swelling, perirectal ulcer or abscess, jaundice, abdominal pain, or abdominal swelling resulting from ascites or a palpable mass [13,14]. Non-Hodgkin's lymphoma can also present with fever, nightsweats, and weight loss which are identical to the constitutional symptoms associated with other AIDS-related disorders. Specific signs which should lead to tissue biopsy (Fig. 11.2) are non-healing perirectal ulcers and/or abscesses, organomegaly with or without ascites, abdominal masses and retroperitoneal lymphadenopathy.

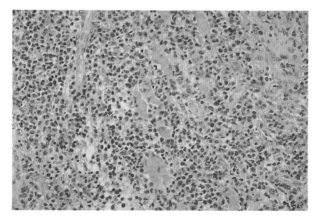

Figure 11.2   Biopsy of anal ulcer featuring small round cells consistent with immunoblastic lymphoma.

Diagnosis of gastrointestinal non-Hodgkin's lymphoma

Non-invasive imaging studies can be useful in identifying suspected NHL, although tissue evaluation is always required to establish the diagnosis. Computerized tomographic (CT) scanning and gallium scans are particularly useful in determining the extent of tumor. Endoscopic biopsies are necessary for the diagnosis of rectal or GI tract tumors. Elevated serum levels of lactate dehydrogenase (LDH) and vric acid are important clues that the patient has NHL.

Treatment

Although various treatment protocols have been employed, most regimens have shown a median survival of only 5–6 months. In fact, two studies have shown that more aggressive chemotherapy regimens have a higher morbidity and mortality. This is due to the development of life-threatening opportunistic infections and poor bone marrow reserve which leads to frequent hospitalizations for fever and neutropenia and chemotherapy does reductions and delays. While overall survival times in patients with AIDS-associated NHL are disappointing, subgroups of patients can be identified in which the therapeutic outcome is significantly better than for other groups of patients. Predictors of good clinical outcome from the San Francisco general series include: CD4+ cells >100 mm^3, no prior diagnosis of AIDS, Karnofsky score of >70%, and no extranodal sites of disease.

Several approaches have been suggested for the treatment of HIV-related lymphomas. These include: use of low doses of chemotherapy, use of high-dose chemotherapy with the addition of GM-CSF or G-CSF, and the use of prophylaxis for pneumocystis. In a study completed through the ACTG, low-dose modification of the m-BACOD regimen had an overall response rate of 51% with a complete response rate of 46% [15]. However, complications included the development of opportunistic infections and neutropenia. In a study performed at San Francisco General Hospital, use of

CHOP was employed either alone or in combination with GM-CSF. The addition of GM-CSF resulted in improvement in hematologic parameters, fewer dose reductions, fewer hospital days, and fewer episodes of febrile neutropenia. However, this was accompanied by some toxicity and included fatigue, diarrhea, fever, and headache. While the development of complete remissions was the same in both groups, the durability of response still needs to be determined. Optimal treatment still has not been determined. In selecting therapy for HIV-associated NHL, the emphasis should be on an individualized treatment. While standard treatment may be appropriate for the patient with good immune function and without a prior opportunistic infection, a lower-dose treatment regimen might be selected for the patient with more severe immune compromise, marginal Karnofsky performance score, and history of opportunistic infections.

Hodgkin's disease

Despite numerous reports suggesting an association of Hodgkin's disease (HD) with the acquired immunodeficiency syndrome, HD in an individual seropositive for the human immunodeficiency syndrome still is not considered a criterion for the diagnosis of AIDS. We recently reported on 23 new cases of HD in individuals at risk for AIDS and reviewed the literature [16,17]. As a group, individuals at risk for AIDS who developed HD had a more aggressive form of the illness (82% with stage III or IV), had or developed AIDS-related opportunistic infections (54%), second neoplasms (10%), and/or profound cytopenias (32%). The tumors were frequently extranodal with frequent involvement of the GI tract; the higher stage was due in large measure to bone marrow involvement by HD, which was present at diagnosis in 48% of patients at risk for AIDS, in contrast to only 3.5% of 659 historical controls.

The single most important factor that limited treatment was the presence or development of neutropenia. More than two-thirds of the patients were dead within one year of the diagnosis of HD. A poor prognosis is associated with fewer than 200 CD4+ cells/mm^3, a prior or concurrent history of an opportunistic infection, and the presence of constitutional symptoms. We conclude that HIV infection alters the clinical course of HD and that advanced or high-grade HD in HIV infected individuals should be considered indicative of AIDS. Optimal treatment still needs to be defined. A study designed to examine the natural history of HD in HIV-positive individuals and examine the toxicity and efficacy of ABVD alone and in combination with GM-CSF is underway through the ACTG.

Squamous cell cancer of the anal region

Epidemiology and etiology
Carcinomas of the anal region represent a rare group of neoplasms accounting for less than 4% of all tumors of the distal gastrointestinal tract. The age-

adjusted risk of carcinoma of the anus and anal canal is 0.6 per 100 000 people each year. In most series the sex incidence for tumors in this region is approximately equal; however, tumors of the anal canal are more common in women, and carcinomas of the anal margin are found more frequently in men. The median age at diagnosis was 65 years, in a review of the incidence of this disease in the USA from 1973 to 1977 [18].

More recently it has become apparent that homosexual men have an increased risk of anal cancer [19] and it is being diagnosed with increased frequency in patients with AIDS. The increased incidence of anal carcinoma in homosexual men suggests that trauma or a venereally transmissible agent may be important factors in pathogenesis. It is possible that the herpex simplex virus and human papillomavirus, which are now considered etiological agents in carcinoma of the cervix, may also play a significant role in the development of anal and perianal carcinoma.

Pathology, diagnosis and staging

The majority of primary anal canal cancers (about 80%) are epidermoid carcinomas, and according to the World Health Organization classification [20] they are subdivided into squamous cell carcinomas (70–80%), transitional, basaloid or cloacogenic carcinomas (20–30%), and mucoepidermoid carcinomas (1–5%). The remainder of anal carcinomas include adenocarcinomas, basal cell carcinomas and melanomas. From a practical point of view, squamous cell carcinomas and transitional or cloacogenic carcinomas have a similar pattern of behavior and prognosis and are managed in a similar way.

The physical investigations should include a digital rectal examination, anoscopy and rectoscopy and a careful evaluation of the inguinal lymph node bearing areas. The presence of metastatic disease in the inguinal lymph nodes should be confirmed with a needle aspiration biopsy or simple excision. Very frequently groin lymph node enlargement is due to reactive hyperplasia and occasionally to the synchronous presence of Kaposi's sarcoma or lymphoma in patients with AIDS.

The recommended staging system to be used is the one described by the UICC or the International Union Against Cancer [21]. This system classifies the primary tumor as a T1 if it is 2 cm or smaller, T2 from 2 to 5 cm, T3 if more than 5 cm in greatest dimension, and T4 when there is invasion of adjacent pelvic organs. The staging of the regional lymph nodes includes the perirectal, internal iliac and inguinal nodal groups.

Management in the non-HIV-infected patient

In 1974, Nigro and coworkers [22] described a preoperative protocol combining simultaneous chemotherapy and radiation therapy in the treatment of anal canal carcinomas. A relatively modest dose of radiation was given (3000 cGy in 15 treatments) with concomitant 24-hour infusion of 5-FU for 5 days plus a single bolus dose of mytomicin C. A 74% rate of tumor control in patients with squamous cell carcinoma of the anus was obtained. Subsequently, other investigators [23–25] have improved these results, using increased amounts of chemotherapy and higher doses of external irradiation.

At the present time, we believe that multimodality therapy including simultaneous chemotherapy and irradiation is the treatment of choice for squamous cell carcinomas of the anus and anal canal. However, the optimal sequencing for chemotherapy and irradiation, the dose time-factors of irradiation and the best combination of chemotherapy agents are not well established owing to the lack of prospective randomized clinical trials.

Our treatment program is similar to the one advocated by John and coworkers in 1987 [25]. Chemotherapy consists of two courses of 5-FU and mytomicin C given simultaneously during the first and last week of the radiation therapy course. 5-FU is given by continuous intravenous infusion for 4 days at a dose of 1000 mg/m^2. Mytomicin C is given by intravaneous bolus on day 1 at the beginning of each 5-FU infusion at a dose of 15 mg/m^2. Radiation is delivered to the primary and regional pelvic lymph nodes utilizing parallel opposing anterior and posterior shaped fields. A total dose of 3060 cGy is given in 17 treatments, followed by a cone-down boost of 1080 cGy to the primary lesion in six treatments. Daily doses of 180 cGy are delivered five times per week. The entire treatment course last 4½ weeks if no treatment interruptions are necessary.

This treatment program has been extremely effective in controling the vast majority of carcinomas of the anus and anal canal, both early and locally advanced. John *et al.* [25] were able to obtain a complete response rate of 86% in 22 patients with the above treatment program. Thus, for the majority of patients a permanent colostomy can be avoided with an excellent disease-free survival. Patients who fail this combination regimen can be salvaged with surgery, either local excision if feasible or abdominoperineal resection. Additional courses of radiation and chemotherapy has been successfully used as salvage treatment in selected patients who failed the initial radiation/chemotherapy regimen without resorting to radical surgery [25].

Management in the HIV infected patient

Our preliminary experiences in the treatment of squamous cell carcinoma of the anal region in patients with AIDS have been rather disappointing. We have recently treated three cases, all homosexual males, with a prior history of multiple partners and anal intercourse. Two patients were staged as T2 and one patient as T3 according to the UICC staging system. Inguinal nodes were palpable in only one case; however biopsy of these nodes revealed Kaposi's sarcoma. CT scans of the pelvis were performed in each case, and no enlarged regional pelvic lymph nodes were visualized. All three patients required multiple interruptions in the radiation therapy course for various periods of time because of marked leukopenia and thrombocytopenia. Furthermore, the second course of chemotherapy had to be delayed for the same reason. Severe diarrhea and electrolyte imbalance was common, requiring hospitalization in two patients. An unusually high degree of early acute perineal dermatitis was seen in all three cases. During the second course of chemotherapy, the dose of mytomicin C had to be reduced by 30% in all three patients, because of persistent pancytopenia.

The inability to treat these patients without interruptions and modifications in the chemotherapy regimen may be one of the reasons for the lack of tumor control in all three patients. In addition, the compromised immune system in this group of patients may have also contributed in some degree to the high failure rate. Although marked regression of the primary lesions was evident during and following completion of the treatment protocol, positive biopsies revealed persistent disease at various time intervals.

This decrease in normal tissue tolerance exhibited by patients with AIDS has been recognized previously by Nisce *et al.* [26] and by Watkins *et al.* [27] who described enhanced mucosal reactions in patients receiving oropharyngeal irradiation for Kaposi's sarcoma. It appears that this lowered normal tissue tolerance may include bowel mucosa and bone marrow as well, most likely because of a defect in the ability of these patients to repair sub-lethal radiation damage.

Other malignancies

Given the large number of individuals infected with HIV in the USA, other problems including other malignancies are to be expected. It may be difficult to establish a direct relationship of these other cancers to HIV infection, but there is a growing suspicion that a relationship may exist. In addition to Kaposi's sarcoma and non-Hodgkin's lymphomas, other cancers have been seen in HIV-positive individuals, including squamous cell carcinomas of the head and neck and rectum, testicular carcinomas of all histologies, malignant melamonas, primary hepatocellular carcinomas, cervical carcinomas, and adenocarcinomas of the lung, stomach, small bowel, colon and rectum. In general, patients without a prior opportunistic infection respond well to aggressive treatment, while individuals with prior opportunistic infections, with fewer than 100 CD4+ cells/mm³, or the presence of severe constitutional symptoms, do poorly (CE Metroka unpublished observations). Recently, attention has been focused on male homosexuals who have evidence of immune dysfunction and a high prevalence of anal human papillomavirus infection and anal intraepithelial neoplasia [28]. It was suggested that as more therapies are available to improve survival, these individuals may be at significant risk for the development of anal cancer.

References

1. Vilmer C, Rouzious C, Vezinet-Brun F, *et al.* Isolation of a new lymphotropic retrovirus from two siblings with Haemophilia B, one with AIDS. *Lancet* 1984; 1:753–7.
2. Gallo RC, Salahuddin SZ Popovic M, *et al.* Frequent defection and isolation of cytopathic retroviruses (HTLV-III) from patients with AIDS and at risk for AIDS. *Science* 1984; **224**:500–3.
3. Nakamura S, Salahuddin Z, Biberfeld, *et al.* Kaposi's sarcoma cells: long term

culture with growth factor from retrovirus-infected CD4+ T cells. *Science* 1988; **242**:242–30.

4. Salahuddin SZ, Nakamura, S, Biberfeld P, *et al.* Angiogenic properties of Kaposi's sarcoma-derived cells after long-term culture *in vitro. Science* 1988; **242**:430–3.

5. Ensoli B, Nakamura S, Salahuddin SZ, *et al.* AIDS–Kaposi's sarcoma-derived cells express cytokines with autocrine and paracrine growth effecs. *Science* 1989; **243**:223–6.

6. Vogel J, Hinrichs SH, Reynolds RK, Luciw PA, Jay G. The HIV tat gene induces dermal lesions resembling Kaposi's sarcoma in transgenic mice. *Nature* 1988; **335**:606–11.

7. Friedman-Kien AE, Saltzman BR, Cao Y, Nestor MS, Mirabile M, Li J. Kaposi's sarcoma in HIV-negative homosexual men. *Lancet* 1990; **i**:168–9.

8. Lifson AR, Darrow WW, Hessol NA, *et al.* Kasposi's sarcoma in a cohort of homosexual and bisexual men: epidemiology and analysis for cofactors. *Am J Epidemiol* 1990; **131**:221–31.

9. Friedman S, Wright T, Altman D. Gastrointestinal manifestations of Kaposi's sarcoma in acquired immunodeficiency syndrome: endoscopic and autopsy findings. *Gastroenterology* 1985; **89**:102–8.

10. Krown SE, Metroka CE, Wernz JC. Kaposi's sarcoma in the acquired immunodeficiency syndrome: a proposal for uniform evaluation, response, and staging criteria. *J. Clin Oncol* 1989; **7**:1201–7.

11. Foong A, Kotler DP, Winkler WP, Pollack J, Metroka CE. Endoscopic laser therapy of obstructing Kaposi's sarcoma. Submitted for publication.

12. Ziegler JL, Beckstead JA, Volberding PA, *et al.* Non-Hodgkin's lymphoma in 90 homosexual men. *New Engl J Med* 1984; **311**:565–70.

13. Ioachim HL, Weinstein MA, Robbins RD, Sohn N, Lugo PN. Primary anorectal lymphoma: a new manifestation of the acquired immune deficiency syndrome. *Cancer* 1987; **60**:1449–53.

14. Burkes RL, Meyer PR, Gill PS, *et al.* Rectal lymphoma in homosexual men. *Arch Intern Med* 1986; **146**:913–5.

15. Levine AM, Wernz JC, Kaplan L, *et al.* Low dose chemotherapy with central nervous system prophylaxis and azidothymidine maintenance in AIDS-related lymphoma: a prospective multi-institutional trial. Submitted for publication.

16. Ames ED, Conjalka MS, Goldberg AF, *et al.* Hodgkin's disease and AIDS: new cases and literature review (abstract). *IVth International Conference on AIDS*, 1988; **2**:no. 2660.

17. Ames ED, Conjalka MS, Goldberg AF, *et al.* Hodgkin's disease and AIDS: twenty-three new cases and a review of the literature. Submitted for publication.

18. Young JL, Percy CI, Asine AJ. *Surveillance, Epidemiology and End Results: Incidence and Mortality Data 1973–1977.* National Cancer Institute Monograph 57, 1981.

19. Peters RK, Mack TM, Bernstein L. Parallels in the epidemiology of selected anogenital carcinomas. *J Nat Cancer Inst* 1984; **72**:609.

20. Morson BC, Sobin JG. Histological typing of intestinal tumors. *International Histological Classification of Tumors*, no. 15. Geneva: World Health Organization, 1976.

21. Harmer MH (ed). *TNM Classification of Malignant Tumors*, 3rd edn. Geneva: Union Internationale Contre le Cancer, 1978.

22. Nigro ND, Vaitkevicius VK, Considine B. Combined therapy for cancer of the anal canal: a preliminary report. *Dis Col Rectum* 1974; **17**:354–6.

23. Cummings B, Keane T, Thomas G, Harwood A, Rider W. Results and toxicity of the treatment of anal canal carcinoma by radiation therapy or radiation therapy and chemotherapy. *Cancer* 1984; **54**: 2062–8.

24. Sischy B. The use of radiation therapy combined with chemotherapy in the

management of squamous cell carcinoma of the anus and marginally resectable adenocarcinoma of the rectum. *Int J Rad Oncol Biol Phys* 1985; **11**:1587–93.

25. John MH, Flam M, Lovalvo L. Mowry AP. Feasability of non-surgical definitive management of anal canal carcinoma. *Int J Rad Oncol Biol Phys* 1987; **13**:299–303.
26. Nisce LF, Safai B. Radiation therapy of Kaposi's sarcoma in AIDS: Memorial Sloan Kettering experience. *Front Radiat Ther Oncol* 1985; **19**:133–7.
27. Watkins EB, Findlay, P, Gelmann E, Lane HC, Zabell A. Enhanced mucosal reactions in AIDS patients receiving oropharyngeal irradiation. *Int J Rad Oncol Biol Phys* 1987; **13**:1403–8.
28. Palefsky JM, Gonzalez J. Greenblatt RM, Ahn DK, Hollander H. Anal intra-epithelial neoplasia and anal papillomavirus infection among homosexual males with group IV HIV disease. *JAMA* 1990; **263**:2911–6.

Index